BACKACHE

Putting It Behind You

Withdrawn

BACKACHE

Putting It Behind You

A spine surgeon discusses advances in rehabilitation and the information that he wishes he had time to tell every patient.

Mark R. Foster, Ph.D., M.D., F.A.C.S.

Rutledge Books, Inc.

Danbury, CT

Interior design by Sharon Gelfand

Cover design by Elizabeth Mihaltse

Rutledge Books, Inc.
107 Mill Plain Road, Danbury, CT 06811
1-800-278-8533
www.rutledgebooks.com

Manufactured in the United States of America
Mark R. Foster
   Backache: Putting It Behind You

ISBN: 1-58244-154-5

   1. Better back health. 2. Latest technologies. 3. Preventative Strategies.

Library of Congress Control Number: 2001090967

Contents

Preface

Listen to the patients, they are trying to tell you the diagnosis.
—Sir William Osler, father of modern medicine

Patients who go to a doctor's office for the problem of low back pain usually take little consolation from the fact that most sufferers of low back pain fully resume their lives, no matter how severe their pain once had been. Perhaps most are not aware of how commonly this problem actually occurs. When socially asked, "How are you?" we do not expect our friends or acquaintances to respond with a list of all the physical woes that they are experiencing at the moment, including headaches, backaches, or other personal problems. In fact, when we have aches or pains, we anticipate that they will go away. If they persist or are severe in our estimation, we call the doctor to discover the cause for persistence or unexpected severity and expect to have an xray or some other diagnostic procedure. Patients with backache expect that a sprain or strain should be like a sprain or strain of the wrist, knee, or ankle, which gets better within days to weeks, causes temporary inconvenience, and is soon forgotten. Most backaches actually do conform with that concept and go away within a few weeks. However, when the pain is severe and, particularly, when the doctor uses this same terminology—sprain or strain—that diagnosis lacks credibility. We went to that doctor because it was not going away, as we expected a sprain or strain would, and that seems to violate our intuition. And further, it now can cause considerable anxiety! Patients want to be certain that they have fully conveyed to the physician all of the problems encountered, how bad it really is, and that the physician has taken the time to analyze their specific case sufficiently in detail to get it right!

The problem is further complicated when a back pain sufferer recognizes not only the matter of pain, but also of the things that he or she is unable to do. When you come to grips with the inability to enjoy leisure activities or even to continue your occupation, then you are going to the doctor not for the pain, but for the disability, and this makes the problem absolutely unacceptable, as we are threatened with an inability to continue our expectations of work, career, and pursuit of recreation.

As a spine surgeon, I have been frustrated with my inability to take sufficient time to really discuss these issues, which are of such momentous concern to my patients. Partly, this is because so much information is available. Also, other patients are already present in the office and waiting to see me and may not accept the fact that they are not just waiting for the physician (who is there and working) but they are also waiting for the patient to whom their physician is currently listening or talking. It is not always possible to anticipate when a particular patient will need substantially more time than is customarily scheduled. Fortunately, many of the questions I hear are voiced repeatedly. For those concerns, I have developed illustrations and some understandable answers and am taking that necessary time to go through the full story about someone's aching back.

Some of this is new, even to many doctors or other health professionals. We have come to recognize that the back is like other parts of the body and, for example, prolonged bed rest is a mistake. For backache, many patients have a fear of doing anything without the doctor's blessing or approval; they will try to walk on a sprained ankle and see how it does or they will try to use the wrist, elbow, or the knee. The back should not be treated differently. Despite severe pain, it may be a sprain that will resolve. Significant advances in rehabilitation, particularly with current evaluation and treatment methods, provides even greater optimism that people will be able to return to their workplace, their occupation, as well as their lives including recreational activities, and we have devoted considerable space to these topics as an update. Just as some teeth will have cold sensitivity after the dentist fixes them, and some ankles will not feel fully normal even after we can run and resume sports, and many aches and pains are just a matter of the aging process, we should be able to resume our lives, our work, and our avocations even though we may not be completely pain free.

Patients want answers but seldom find satisfactory or convincing information, or more importantly, feel heard or even believed. With a comprehensive back-care program, this can be a reassuring story, particularly for the category of patient who truly has a problem and needs detailed care, information, and treatment, but would not benefit from surgical intervention. These people are often left in limbo, as they may seek a surgeon or are referred by their family doctor as a failure of conservative (nonsurgical) care, and then when the surgeon says they don't need surgery, they have no place left to turn.

Congratulations! You do not need an operation. You then ask, "What should I do? How can I proceed with my disrupted life and plans?" At that point, the surgeon is done. The opinion is issued. As captain of the ship and head of the totem pole, the sufferer wants his further opinion on what is best to do now, but that does not follow—if the surgeon cares for all the nonsurgical cases, when will he be able to operate? This is frustrating and not immediately reasonable to the person stuck with pain that no one could fix, hence the referral to the surgeon!

This book is to help you understand what the surgeon might say if he could take the time. It is written specifically to provide information that will make all of the treatments and expectations of medical or other treatments understandable. It is in a specific order so, barring my failure to make it nontechnical and understandable to the lay person, what you will need to be able to understand the material anywhere in the text should be presented in the pages preceding and thus be self-contained. To those physicians or other health-care professionals who may elect to read this book, please feel free to use any of the illustrations or explanations which may be of assistance to you in explaining this information to your patients.

—M.R.F.

Chapter 1

PERSPECTIVE

Examination. If thou examinest a man having a sprain of the vertebra of his spinal column, thou shouldst say to him: extend thou your legs and contract them both. He contracts them both immediately because of the pain he causes in the vertebra of the spinal column in which he suffers. Diagnosis. Thou shouldst say to him: one having a sprain in the vertebra of his spinal column, an ailment I shall treat. Treatment. Thou shouldst place him prostrate on his back . . .

—Edwin Smith,
Papyrus 1500 B.C.

Low back pain has a very long and distinguished history from which perhaps we can better understand the situation. Egyptian mummies have been shown to have degenerative changes, as have the spines of the earliest remains of Neanderthals. The Egyptians apparently treated with bed rest the afflictions of the spine, and so does Western medicine traced back to Hippocrates. Sciatica was understood by Hippocrates and when it radiated to the foot, it was considered good; if it remained only in the hip, it was dreaded. This fear was engendered by the lack of expectation of relief, not because it was more severe, as it was actually less severe, but because the end was not in sight. Sciatica was customarily an affliction lasting about forty days and thought to be an excess of cold. (Now we customarily treat for six weeks, or forty-two days!) Hence, the remedy was local heat provided by spas, ointments, and counterirritants. The Greeks considered back pain as a fleeting symptom of joints and muscles, and also incorporated the use of spas and soothing local applications of counterirritants.

Rheumatism was prominent in the seventeenth century, where the Greek *rheuma*, a watery discharge of evil humor flowing from the brain, was thought to cause pain in the joints or other parts of the body. Rheumatism was thought to be caused or worsened by exposure to cold and damp, and specifically, trauma was excluded as an inciting cause. In the nineteenth century, the idea of spinal nerve irritation arose and became popular, even though the pathology was not yet identified. It was subsequent, in the latter half of the nineteenth century, when the Industrial Revolution and the building of railways led to serious injuries, that opinion gradually evolved to consider that chronic back pain (railway spine) could be the result of cumulative trauma, as well as the crippling injuries from sudden severe catastrophic injury and the recognition of compensation through the Railway Act and laws arising from the building of the railway system.

The principles of bed rest for orthopedic injuries were not restricted to back pain but were strongly advocated in the nineteenth century. Bones were thought to heal reliably when held in a plaster of Paris cast. Consistent with this philosophy, patients with back pain were kept at bed rest, enforced and prolonged. Unfortunately, joints are meant to move. We now understand and universally accept the concept that following injuries to the joints, in most cases, the injured area should be mobilized as soon as possible. Often this is accomplished by the performance of open reduction, surgically stabilizing the bony injury with an internal fixation device; for example, using rods or plates and screws with other various devices, so that joint motion can be restored early and muscles start acting. The modern era of operating and using internal fixation for bony injury has allowed restoration of normal function in adjacent joints, which would have with earlier treatments resulted in healed bones but with stiff and dysfunctional joints, if kept in a plaster cast for prolonged proscribed periods.

From a historical standpoint, this perspective needs to be appreciated because the idea of prolonged bed rest for the back, contrary to the remainder of the body, does persist to the modern day, even though studies have shown that it does not help further (and may even be counterproductive,) for backaches after about two days' time. Nonetheless, prolonged enforced bed rest has not been abandoned in many cases. It is interesting that many of the basic principles of Orthopedics were well stated by Sir John Thomas in England, whose father was a bonesetter or manipulator, and thus had roots historically similar to a chiropractor. Departing from his father's trade and becoming an orthopedic surgeon, we observe a stark contrast. Early mobilization by the bonesetters was not viewed with any moderation, but reacted against with vigor. Patients were routinely advised to lie down when their back ached with the expectation that it would cure all pain and subsequently they could gradually resume activities. This is not the case for an injured knee, wrist, shoulder, or elbow. Those joints need to be moved, as we now understand that nutrition to the articular cartilage, as well as the disc, is dependent upon joint motion. Further, the use of the muscles surrounding the joint as early as possible is necessary to minimize muscular atrophy, which is not entirely reversible. Clearly, for the case of a frozen shoulder, relief of pain is recognized to be dependent upon reachieving full motion of the joint. The analogy is obvious to the back and to back pain, but is not widely appreciated even by some professionals in the field.

With the Industrial Revolution and particularly the building of railroads, lumbago as a major cause of disability grew and became possible with the development of a social support system, in terms of compensation for workers. The industrial back problem became a major concern in the first several decades of the twentieth century with efforts concentrated on better diagnosis and treatment, as well as better detection of malingering (pretending to be ill or incapacitated to escape work or receive benefits). Subsequent attention was turned to the better selection of employees and the improvement of working practices to prevent injuries with this common and expensive problem. At this early stage, back pain was considered a fitness problem rather than a medical problem and efforts at rehabilitation were started. Most disability was listed as rheumatism, exceeded only by insanity, as the principal cause of inability to work in younger people.

The problem of low back pain is almost ubiquitous and some have recommended that it be considered normal in human experience. It is in many cases a nuisance phenomenon and was considered an illness, not an injury, until recently, particularly since the time of the Industrial Revolution. That is, patients who had pain in their back had lumbago, presuming that the quadratus lumborum was responsible, and hence the diagnosis was of a muscular problem—lumbago. There was no diagnostic proof that the quadratus lumborum was involved, and certainly there are many cases today where pain is located specifically in that area and may, in fact, be the quadratus lumborum syndrome of historical interest, but is almost never identified as such today.

Anatomic descriptions of the intervertebral disc and the facet joints in the middle nineteenth century were available, but not commonly connected to the disease of low back pain or radiating leg pain. In particular, cases had been reported of major trauma injuring a disc and causing pain, but until the twentieth century and the newly emerging specialty of spine surgery, which began to consider the severe cases leading to sciatica and cauda equina syndrome (paralysis with loss of bowel and bladder function), the idea that benign cartilaginous tumors or enchondromas of the spinal canal might benefit from surgical intervention remained dominant. Hence, the pain in the back or radiation down the leg, which might be associated with these cartilaginous masses or enchondromas, should perhaps have been considered a result of the reported cases of major trauma, but back pain remained generally a fitness problem and was not considered or attributed to trauma or an industrial accident. Our present task is to find the appropriate balance between the earliest concept that everything was a problem with fitness, to the more recent extreme of emphasizing only the compensable injury, so that we can maximally rehabilitate and restore the injured person to greatest productivity and lifestyle. With heart disease, exercise is prescribed with active patient involvement; with back pain, the prescription of disability or work restrictions and generally passive treatments (done to the patient) are prescribed. There is considerable denial on the part of most working men that they are not as fit as they were when they were nineteen, but fitness is a matter of degree and professional athletes are not expected to function until they are sixty-five. We need to accept the fact that fitness is clearly a part of the problem, contributing to the prolonged need for extensive treatment, even in cases where there was absolutely no pain prior to the incident or injury when the disability originated. No one would ever fault Larry Bird of the Boston Celtics for lack of initiative or ever giving less than his total effort; however, his back failed before he was forty.

In the early 1920s, the sacroiliac joint that was blamed for most low back pain. This may have been because of the appearance of sacroiliac sur-

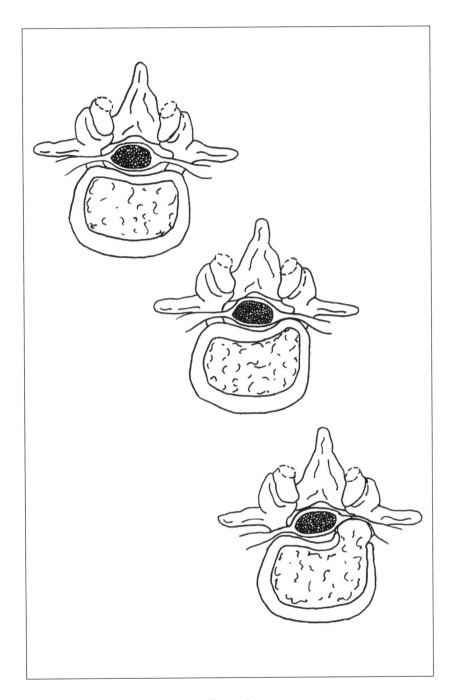

Figure 1

Normal, bulging, and herniated disc.

gery, the arthrodesis (fusion operation). In addition to sacroiliac manipulation, sacroiliac belts, or other appliances were available for treatment, so a
problem was sought to make best use of these solutions. This dramatically
changed in the 1930s when a patient at the Massachusetts General Hospital
was operated on for what was then first recognized to be a rupture of a portion of the inner part (nucleus) of a disc rather than a chondroma or tumor
of the disc. This patient had suffered previous trauma and neurologic findings had been treated nonsurgically for years with little success. After surgery, he was much improved, although the recommendation which suggested that a fusion accompany the disc surgery, is still controversial.

This ushered in the "Dynasty of the Disc" where many have just looked
upon people with low back pain and said, "It's from the disc." Figure 1
(page 5) shows a normal, bulging, and a ruptured disc, in which the ruptured portion is near a nerve root and could understandably cause pressure
on that root with subsequent pain down the leg into the area served by that
nerve root. Recognizing that this nerve serves the muscle of the foot and sensation in that area, we need to clearly understand that back pain is not
explained by pressure of this nerve, and that the general concept of having
a disc rupture generally refers to pressure on the nerve to the foot (sciatica)
which is inconsistent with back pain; that is, pain in the back may be from
aging or deterioration of the disc without pressure on the nerve. Not only
was back pain not the reason that the disc was operated on in the 1930s, it
also should not be the reason to operate on a herniated disc today. Patients
with a ruptured disc may have the pressure of the jelly escaping from the
doughnut, as the disc is often viewed, but a ruptured disc speaks of some of
the jelly outside of the doughnut offending the nerves and causing leg pain.
We will discuss at length in the following chapters the complex situation of
the structures in the back and try to explain the origin of the pain.

When we consider Third World countries, we find that low back pain
is very common, but actual disability cannot arise even with the introduction of modern medicine until a social system is installed. Patients are crippled by falling out of trees and breaking their backs, as well as by tubercu-
losis or polio, but no one is prescribed bed rest to interrupt their activity, or
is permanently disabled by the onset of simple low back pain. This has been
documented by Dr. Gordon Waddell in studies in Oman, where the lives of

individuals are not complicated by a social system that seeks to guarantee a certain standard of living or continuity of income which cannot be interrupted by injury on the job; people do what they can. Perhaps a difference in perspective or expectation exists, as disease may take the lives of their children, they may die of illnesses treatable elsewhere, they may go blind from simple bacterial infections, the most common cause of blindness in the world, and retirement is not their shared dream. Hence, litigation is not available to remedy these economic losses, they are forced to accept whatever they have already earned but have no claim on the future or their anticipations. Conversely, they may not have mortgage payments and revolving credit installments attached to the promise of their anticipated paychecks.

To illustrate, I recall suffering the loss of a very dear automobile (the first new car that I had purchased, which was totaled in an accident). I had felt assuredly that my car would provide enjoyment beyond mere transportation for many years to come. Without physical pain, except perhaps for the first week after the accident, I suffered a loss of expectations, of long-established camaraderie, and was not well compensated by my insurance for the vehicle. Nonetheless, my payment was final and I had to replace the vehicle in any way that I desired. When a worker has a physical injury, we realize that suffering and the inability to work are far more complex than simply an injury to muscles, the discs, or any other structures in the spine. Suffering the loss of that first new automobile brought into my mind my independence and youth, the passing of which was difficult to accept, particularly as the vehicle had not depreciated in my mind to the extent in actual fact that it had lost considerable value and function.

The situation becomes an extremely complex matter, as suffering is actually a matter of behavior, and the inability to work is not solely a physical concern, but combinations of perceptions and experiences of each individual, and their response to these situations which determine the outcome. If we consider a paraphrase of a statement by Henry Wadsworth Longfellow, we see ourselves in terms of our dreams or expectations whereas others see us in terms of our accomplishments. There certainly are losses that we may suffer that are not provable or demonstrable and hence not compensable. That is, we expect certain things to come about and if an accident changes our path so that we cannot accomplish what we had planned, we may be forced to recognize that plans and hope are not assets; they are not yet accomplishments. Our viewpoint seems only reasonable to us, but it doesn't seem at all reasonable when we present it to someone who is paying the bill. We find it distressing, not only that they do not accept our calculation of our losses, but also the payer does not even see the basis on which we are computing what we would have been able to do (loss of opportunity) had it not been for the injury. To state this another way, we should look at human illness rather than specific disease, from a holistic view of medicine. This better describes disability as being "unfit" for work, as opposed to considering the pain (or particularly chronic pain) which makes us ill and the pain then causes disability. If we see ourselves as unfit for a particular work, we would naturally seek other work, unless someone is responsible. In that case, we would then collect the same salary from the person responsible for causing the injury to us, as we would if we had continued on that job. The difference is that we are not producing any usable work when we are out of work. Many patients fill in my initial questionnaire regarding their employment as "disability." It has always been interesting to me that no one is really hiring for that job, but a lot of people feel that it is their bonafide description of their employment.

To return to the analogy, I had to accept the loss of a relatively old car, which still seemed fairly new to me, and was forced to find other transportation. After a significant motor vehicle accident, even after you sign off with the body shop for the repair, if you ever sell that car you will become acutely aware of the loss in value because it has been in an accident. Many patients seem to have an attitude along that line—how will I find any other work after I have sustained a back injury? It may be possible for me to do my job, but it hurts and it did not hurt before. What restitution is there for this pain that I am suffering? Patients who sustain an industrial injury need to accept the fact that things are different; they are not likely to be restored to their expectations and dreams (as I did not immediately return to a new car as I was a medical student at the time). We have to recognize the complexity of the problem, and with the help of the coordinated resources of an appropriate team of rehabilitation professionals, we should be able to assess what we can do as we face the future for our maximal best interests and enjoyment of life, career, and recreation. Outcomes in patients who are on disability for the same disease or same indications for surgery or for the same nonsurgical treatment, particularly without the appropriate comprehensive facilities that are often needed, are not as good as they are in other patients not on disability with the same physical problems.

Unfortunately in some of these cases, the patients are treated by the insurance carrier and even the physicians and perhaps mostly by fellow workers, as second-class citizens when in fact these individuals are following well-meaning doctor's orders and are indeed responding to the many factors other than the physical problems that result in the pain in their back, which pain they suffer with great sincerity. Certainly these patients are equally if not more frustrated at their inability to resume productive employment and their place among their fellow workers, as well as their recreational activities. We thus conclude from this perspective that disability is an invention, not of Western medicine, but is a social problem of recent origin, which currently threatens the competitiveness of the United States or even of our Western economy.

This has been such a significant problem, both in terms of expense and suffering, that national conferences have been held. The National Institutes of Health convened a study group in 1988, updating what has become known since their previous study in 1980 and suggesting areas to be researched. The International Society for the Study of the Lumbar Spine meets annually and published a volume in 1990, *The Lumbar Spine*. From this we have a compendium of an enormous amount of information that is published with the specific intent of guiding further research to contribute to this problem. A comprehensive text, *The Adult Spine* was published in 1991 with more than one hundred chapters, and weighs seventeen pounds. With all the information that is known, we certainly must recognize that a great deal is being done for this problem; however, we do not have the solution to all low back pain problems nor have we diminished the enormous number of patients who are suffering from this problem and are on disability.

Labor and industry remain aware of the impact this is having on the international competitiveness of our exports and national products. In our society, we have heard of extremely good results in the care of patients with back pain and particularly some spectacular results with minimally interventional surgeries (microscopes, suction techniques, and lasers).

Hearing of these new techniques, patients may have a problem that is frustrating to them, prevents them from returning to normal activities, and for which they would like to have something done, even surgically, but for which surgical intervention may or may not be appropriate. Certainly not all surgical cases can have the same excellent expectation as the glowing reports that have been heard from friends and coworkers or promoted in the media. This book represents a caveat emptor approach to the low back pain patient who feels that the only solution is surgical; however, we also provide enough detail to explain that there is assistance available for the patient for whom surgery is not indicated and that the massive explosion of information does provide a good functional prognosis for that patient as well.

In recent years the surgery has gotten very specific, minimally invasive, and highly technological, but effectiveness remains completely dependent upon the need of the patient; that is, the most perfect gall bladder operation in the world will not help a patient who has appendicitis. Recognizing the fact that many studies have demonstrated an incidence or occurrence rate of surgically amenable disc problems in less than two-percent of patients with severe low back pain, and thus the pain of the 98 percent, which is often just as severe, only different in its pattern, is not a surgical problem. We thus need to recognize that the majority must be treated without surgical intervention, and subsequently cease the continual tempting of surgeons to lower their indications and expectations by sending all of the severe cases, having failed to respond to the simple, customary, and usual initial treatment within a specified time such as six weeks, for a surgical opinion.

The general physician who sends the patient for a consultation to the cardiologist has to continue treating that patient if the cardiologist says that the problem is not cardiac or surgical in nature. The patient with low back pain who is sent to the spine surgeon expects that expert to solve all of the pain problems, as the referral implies that they know more than the referring physician. It must be recognized that nonsurgical problems can be treated by the nonsurgeon who is interested and informs himself or herself, and further, that the surgeon has special training to do surgery and usually higher overhead costs such as office and malpractice insurance and other matters, which make it unreasonable to expect the person who has restricted practice to surgery to deviate from that specialization election.

Unfortunately, most surgeons give a glib "it will get better" to patients who are referred as a failure of therapy and are not getting better, but these patients do not get a return appointment to tell the doctor that he or she was wrong: it is really not getting better; This lack of clear direction contributes to the illness and disability. Patients come away convinced only that the surgeon does not understand or care, or does not have the talents to handle their particular problem.

We do not expect the obstetrician to take care of the infant child rather than the pediatrician; however, the obstetrician certainly has to have a lot of information prior to the delivery and this physician has to be specifically trained and knowledgeable to ensure the delivery of a healthy infant. There seems to be a lack of perception, not only among the public but among referring physicians, that low back pain is cared for by surgeons even when it is a nonsurgical problem, as they exhibit greater expertise by being able to take care of the surgical or at least in concept more severe cases. The emphasis of this book is to explain the complexity of the problem and the need for an equally comprehensive solution as the severity is excessive in all cases where disability is involved. The problem exceeds the expertise of a single individual, even a surgeon.

Chapter 2

PROBLEM

It ill behooves the skilled physician to mumble charms
over ills that crave the knife.

—Sophocles

A BIG PROBLEM

Back pain is a very common problem. Statistically, 80 percent of people
will lose time from their occupation at some point during their working
career due to a back problem. If misery loves company, then a back problem
is certainly a place where you need not fear being alone. Perhaps there
should be some consolation in the fact, that so many people are affected and
even of those severely affected, most will recover quickly and completely. It
is self-evident from the magnitude of the problem that it is basically not a
surgical problem, and that most people do well without an operation.

This enormous problem is the cause of an enormous expense. The medical
costs come first to mind, but lost wages and productivity far exceed
those costs. As a matter of fact, it is the number one cause of disability for
working people between the ages of twenty and forty. The annual cost
exceeds $100 billion annually and is growing. Approximately a quarter of a
million people undergo surgery for spine problems annually and of these a
significant portion return to work, but some require further surgery and
another fraction never return to productivity or employment.

Although some seem to see it otherwise, the world is not bogged down
by back pain. The present problem is currently out of control and the insurance
carriers may actually be as much disabled by fear of the cumulative
problem, for which they have to project reserves, as is the individual disabled
by fear of pain or other consequences of returning to work and the

inability to project reserves for his or her retirement, leisure, and family needs. Unfortunately, the insurance companies collect a percentage of the money, which goes through their hands from premiums to insured losses; and as the claims rise, the net insurance industry profits also increase as a percentage of the total. Most people who have had a severe episode have returned to completely normal and fully participate in all of their customary activities. In fact, the prognosis is very good; 90 percent of people who have back pain will not seek further medical attention within three months. Although we may take some consolation in the fact that we are in good company and that most people do well, it is truly intimidating to be unable to do customary things, and there is great fear associated with the disability that accompanies low back pain.

The fact that there is a statistically excellent chance that we will recover completely does not diminish the other facts, namely that this is an enormously expensive problem, not only in economic terms, but also in terms of human suffering and disability. It has always seemed to me a paradox that most patients are fearful that they will be disabled by their low back pain and yet they remain convinced that the patients on chronic disability with whom they are familiar are all fakers. I have never forgotten the patient who sat on the examining table and told me not only that he was in pain, but that he was not like all the others—he was actually in pain. He was very puzzled when I suggested to him that I found the others credible—I believed them, and I couldn't understand why he didn't believe them, particularly since he was experiencing pain. My supposition is that, since most people have back pain at some point in their lives or working career, they expect that others have back pain like theirs: troubling but not disabling, something that a real man would tolerate. Having had minor pains, they have concluded that most back pain complainers are wimps or essentially they do not believe their fellow human being's complaints of severe pain as being genuine.

BACK PAIN—NOT ME!

People are forced to deal with this problem which may occur on a very untimely occasion. It is not so much a matter of being unlucky and getting involved by having an episode of back pain, but rather how we handle it and how we prepare ourselves. The fear of becoming disabled and having unrelenting pain without any satisfactory solution medically or surgically cannot be relieved simply with the statistics that I have presented. This brings to mind the statistician who, being of normal height, drowned while crossing a stream with an average depth of three feet. Each individual may after all be one of the 10 percent who do poorly, so the 90 percent, who do well cannot reassure an individual. The fact that this is a benign disease fails to reassure patients who are in pain and unable to do the things that they took for granted, such as continuing at their job, seeking promotions, pursuing leisure activities, and maintaining their current lifestyle. We seem to hold staunchly to the concept that it is our right and the obligation of modern medicine to maintain us pain-free from back problems, even though we accept the fact that we may die from a heart attack or be crippled by arthritis. If we have a lot of contingencies and no reserve for emergencies, then we may have a poor perspective and blame the episode of back pain or another illness or unexpected increased expenses in one month as responsible for all of our plans and aspirations being set back rather than keeping in perspective that we were not prepared to handle eventualities.

I recall with relish an elderly surgeon who was answering questions following a presentation at an international meeting. One person in the audience asked this distinguished gentleman whether or not patients who were treated as he had recommended might have problems "down the road." With minimal pause, and perhaps some condescension, this surgeon stated with considerable emphasis, "We're all going to have problems down the road." From his age and accomplishments, it is likely that he was speaking from personal experience and perhaps felt that he was stating the obvious. Nonetheless, when people present to their doctors with back pain, they are not simply asking how to handle the pain, they are deeply concerned about their inability to do things, as some people cannot do, such as continue to work, enjoy their leisure, and so forth. Back pain has notoriety in terms of causing disability, which precedes it and causes this anxiety.

Perhaps the situation is somewhat analogous to the long-standing love affair between drivers and their automobiles. This is a complex love-hate relationship, but may illustrate the matter at hand. A new car sparkles, is shown off, and of course is justified as getting us "to work." We see some signs a bit later on, "Don't laugh—it's paid for." We understand that after time has passed, the shine will dull and mechanical difficulties will arise. The problem occurs when we encounter the familiar syndrome, namely that we are concerned about breaking down and spending a few hundred dollars in repair bills on a less-than-monthly basis. Hence we promptly go out and buy a new model, and then on a regular basis over an extended period, expend considerably more than those few hundred dollars of repair bills. We rest assured that after we get the "bugs" out, we will be able to drive reliably to work, while we are complaining about the lemon that we were sold. In the meanwhile, we conceal our true enchantment with the shine and newer-than-the-neighbor's-car attitude.

Many patients with whom I converse seem to boast that they don't go to the doctor unless they need to, to telegraph their point to the doctor that they are not being wimpy, as they presume other back pain suffers are, but they have a really severe problem. As a matter of conversation, it seems they are attempting to distinguish themselves from the norm. This, however, seems in fact to be the norm, namely to avoid going to the doctor unless it is necessary. Perhaps this is because illnesses are better covered by insurance than office calls for people who are well, but it also represents a macho sense in which they feel above illness, having been imbued by their Creator with the right of good health. There is, however, no way to collect on that warranty except to present to the health-care practitioner and expect not only restoration, but also assurance that they won't have further problems. The doctor is not amused by this attitude of many, that it is as if the physician were at fault for the pain, or particularly, the lack of immediate and complete relief.

PAIN OR DISABILITY

A similar attitude seems to be prominent in some patients who present with back pain. These individuals may be out of work for only a few days and then feel better; nonetheless, they present to the doctor's office because they don't want to have to deal with that backache again. They emphatically present to the physician the facts, which are namely that they are not sick and, most of all, that they don't come to the doctor all the time for every little thing. This is not to offend the doctor, but to straighten out the physician with the fact that they are really in this case very sick, incapable of their normal schedule, and that this back discomfort is intolerable and must be taken care of definitively. Even though this is a macho attitude, namely of good health, the prescription of exercise and fitness that would seem entirely appropriate for such a healthy individual and commonly prescribed for back problems is not accepted or even is mocked as the physician's failure to understand how healthy they are and how that may commonly be someone else's problem but could not possibly be their problem.

Even though during the course of our employment or other activities, we may spend prolonged periods either sitting, standing, or doing many activities, we do not realize the extent to which other postures of the body are never attained or some motions of the spine are not part of our usual activities, and as such, posture and fitness exercises would be the most appropriate thing to restore a full range of motion and comfort to the spine. The presumption is, because of the pain and other good health, that there must be a drastic problem on the X rays or some study, which another doctor will be able to find, which certainly has to be present since such a healthy and fit person couldn't possibly have a backache so drastically out of keeping with the careful attention to good health, overall motivation and constitution, and self-evident vitality. Unfortunately, this patient, or patient's attitude, is really stacked against the physician. Problems which occur just with aging and are commonly seen on X rays are present in patients without any complaints whatsoever, but may be attributed to their problem by noncritical doctors and chiropractors without any evidence to correlate those X ray findings with the actual complaints. While it is increasingly well known that many patients without any pain whatsoever may have X ray changes of disc degeneration, to have your doctor say that you have a blown-out disc certainly fits the pain you are experiencing and such a graphic description would certainly be expected to require a drastic solution. The patient's mind that is already made up and attempting to excuse these X ray findings as anything less than totally consistent with his disability would seem argumentative and unproductive. Unfortunately, this terminology may label a person, at least in his or her own mind, who was otherwise restorable or rehabilitatable, as diseased in a way that feeds into needing the health professional. That is, the chiropractor who describes severe disc problems will also find the patient willing to undergo a prolonged series of manipulations or the not-very-busy surgeon may have convinced this person that surgery is the only suitable remedy; or, if later the imaging studies do not justify surgery, that any worsening in the future would mean they would have to come back to that particular surgeon for a profitable procedure. X-ray findings of dried out (bulging) discs, a normal aging phenomenon, or other similar findings are present in people without symptoms and may be contributing to symptoms, but the embellishment of those degenerative findings as blown out disc is probably never justified. The patient experiencing pain is also convinced that they may unfortunately need to accept permanent limitations, in terms of lifting or other activities, because of their injured back, and thus a disability is created by the graphic description used rather than the specifics of the spinal pathology, which we will discuss in the next chapter and which is often present in people who are doing heavy work without any symptoms whatsoever.

Many people allegedly go to their doctor because of the pain, but their conversation, if we would actually write down the words and look at them carefully, would reveal that without admitting it, they are really scared of their inability to do various things because of their back pain problem. They go because they really want it taken care of and they want it fixed, almost as if it were warranty work. They want it done promptly, with minimal interference in their activities, and without any extended treatments, because they are otherwise healthy and they take care of themselves or more accurately are too healthy to need to give any attention to their body. If we are unable to tolerate pain, we come to the doctor and expect to be admitted; if we cannot walk, the doctor orders crutches or a wheelchair; if we are not able to work, the doctor writes a slip to keep the utilities from being cut off in the winter; but the compensation system frequently involves patients who are stressed by their case in litigation and realistically the defense intends to cause some economic distress for the purpose of moving the case along, settling, or at least just finding out where they stand in terms of reserves—the doctor's perceived power to relieve all of the stresses and problems that the patient cannot deal with does not extend to this economic arena.

A careful listener will detect considerable conversation and questioning which relates to an underlying tacit concern of whether the back problem will come back again, even though the literature declares that it's a chronic recurrent problem with a 60 percent incidence of another period of disability in patients who have been off and successfully returned to activities, within two years of the initial episode. Perhaps frustration with this component of the problem engenders the desire to be sent to a specialist, even a surgeon, with whom we are not familiar, and particularly, who is not familiar with the patient, the patient's background, or job stresses and so forth that may be integral to the problem.

If there is a problem, certainly the severity would dictate the need to undergo an operation or anything necessary to get rid of the back pain and to prevent joining one of those tragic few who are chronically disabled, always in pain, unable to get satisfactory help (but who we seem to think are faking it, even though we fear becoming one of them). This is not as simple as getting a new battery for our automobile in anticipation of the cold weather when we notice that the old one is not cranking well to start the car in the fall. We will all remain subject to getting the flu, the common cold, or other illnesses (and know that recovery may be slowed by our choice of continuing smoking) and as a consequence, will lose work time perhaps every year, but these problems do not carry the same emotional impact as having a backache.

As a physician, I can confirm the impression that many patients have what could be perhaps paraphrased as, What You Always Wanted to Know About Your Doctor's Attitude Towards Your Backache, But Were Afraid to Ask. This has perhaps contributed to many helpful clips in the media, titled, Ask Your Doctor. This is despite the fact that it is getting increasingly difficult to ask your mechanic what's wrong with your car because he needs a computer diagnostic setup to understand the problem and when he just tells you which components have failed, he has to give you an extended functional description and a basic education on how your car runs for you to understand why that part has caused your particular problem. The doctor has considerable knowledge about your back to which the patient expects a twenty-five-words-or-less explanation. The problem is so severe and the information so captivating when personalized to a patient, that they get fixated on every word that the physician should use. Nonetheless, every word or every anatomic region or body component part has a very intricate function for which the patient has enormous preconceived notions, most of which are oversimplified or even wrong and which cause major confusion. It seems in many cases that the more the doctor tells the patient, the more questions come up and the less the patient understands. My response has been to write this book and hope that it may be understandable and read by as many as are truly interested. In reality, I find most of my explanations dealing with the oversimplified misconceptions that have been used by other physicians to get a customer satisfied and out of the office; that is, the patient is pleased with the explanation even if it is wrong and the doctor has satisfaction from having pleased the patient, and now being able to move forward on his schedule to the next irritated individual who thinks he or she has been waiting too long.

Many patients are merely inquisitive or being conversational and hence the physician may want to avoid "wasting time" on a detailed discussion and hence will say, "It's a disc" or "It's a muscle," or some other explanation. They want to summarily end the discussion first, which is really going no place unless the patient is committed to doing some real studying, and second, because we really don't have a good explanation of the exact origin of the pain which would stand up to scientific analysis. Actually a diagnosis is not truly available in about eighty-percent of cases according to the scientific literature, and studies have identified about fifty different technical terms describing the same condition, the common backache, each having some value and added perspective. Further, we have a responsibility to remain professional and objective about signs and symptoms rather than to become "friends" with a few patients. Being a professional who is compassionate and treats patients in a caring way, is important as long as it does not lessen or compromise our objectivity. The patient is truly not helped by excessively focusing attention on how hard it is to deal with a back problem. The real need is to put it behind us and go forward with what we can do with professional help despite the problem. I often recall my first encounter in an operating room as a volunteer, probably the only Ph.D. mopping floors, and hearing the chief surgeon say to the cardiothoracic resident during an open heart operation, "Stop gawking at such a classic ventriculoseptal defect and sew it up." The hole in that patient's heart exceeded any textbook for interest and detail, but the patient needed to get off the operating table!

Patients who are desperately trying to cope with their problem and find no help from the treatments offered also have found no sympathy from the company or the insurance carrier, so they turn to their physician as a last resort. Unfortunately, the physician cannot categorically say the patient needs help and coerce the insurance carrier into a sympathetic or sometimes even cooperative situation. Rather, the physician has an obligation to relate the diagnosis and other technical information to the adjuster who then decides, or as many have asserted, practices medicine. The unsatisfied patient may seek another physician, still convinced that the doctor can control the situation, and the next physician may sincerely gloss over the problem, but unfortunately pick a different anatomic feature (the disc rather than the muscle or vice versa) and hence the patient can't reconcile the two explanations. Is it really a disc or is it muscles? Did they both believe me or are they both patronizing me? Or does neither understand my problem? Are they just lying to me?

WHAT'S A DOCTOR TO DO?

Doctors are clearly not excited about seeing patients who have low back pain. First of all, many of these patients may have disability and while they are on compensation, they seem to elicit a uniform physician response: the avoidance reflex! Not only are the patients' problems complicated by interference with their recovery from the insurance carrier, who not only delays approval of treatments that should be provided in a timely fashion, but there also is a burdensome amount of paperwork involved in caring for these patients. Further, the physician always gets blamed as the reason they are not getting their disability check. (Why would the doctor want to stop their check, as opposed to the adjuster who wants to cut costs but have the doctor blamed?) Really the doctor is told to put a square peg in a round hole on carefully worded forms that are intended to put the physician on the defensive, as if the doctor was at fault for the patient's inability to function at the workplace, as though the doctor was on trial to prove that the patient can't work. This started with the federal government, where benefits were denied through computer programs looking at codes, which the patient could not enter without the manuals or expertise. The codes essentially treated everyone by the averages when they are on Medicare. So individual exceptions and specific needs were ignored "your doctor" didn't think you needed a certain service according to a letter from the Federal Government to the patient. Meanwhile, the physician, on his own time and at his own expense and with distraction from other patients, is attempting to appeal such a decision. A lot of those denials by "your doctor" are without the doctor's awareness although he is being credited with making the denial. The doctor is also under obligation to enter the code that honestly best represents the situation, and having signed the form that he acknowledges that he will go to jail if it is not the correct code, the computer has declared, as a consequence, that the physician didn't want the patient to be treated in the manner in which the patient felt was appropriate, even though the physician may actually have wanted that specific treatment to be provided.

I recall an international meeting where a judge was asked by a physician, "When the patient is no longer totally disabled, is able to do something, but is not able to return to a job, the doctor is blamed since, the subsequent letter with notification of termination of benefits attributes this to the doctor's report." The judge then harshly and condescendingly told the doctor as if sentencing a convicted criminal, "Just give us the medical doctor." A state senator who was sitting next to the judge, admitted that "priority" assigned to this case still meant that it wasn't heard within twelve weeks and I am sure the judge was not in danger of losing his house or car by missing three payments waiting for the resolution of the situation. The president of this meeting pointed out that to bring some reality to the judge's ivory tower, surgeons have been killed by disgruntled patients after these letters go out from the court evasively saying "your doctor has determined you are no longer totally disabled." That decision is administratively a legal matter and the responsibilities of the court, so why do the judges fail to state that they have decided on the facts. Courts determine facts, doctors determine impairment, and disability is the court's responsibility based on the medical input of the impairment for which the court awards benefits. The fact remains: there is little objectivity to go on, so the decision actually does rest largely on a matter of opinion. The treating doctor's opinion is likely to favor the patient, and the physician selected by the insurance company is selected for bias the other way. Unfortunately, minor differences in opinions within this particular area are without significant objective basis to make a precise decision, and these small differences make an enormous difference for the patient.

Physicians are not eager, having been through medical school, to become a clerk for the cataloging, and to provide ad nauseam, a description of activities that cause the patient pain, and then be told that they are subjective, as if inconsequential, at least to the insurance company, or legally, which then becomes the basis for the patient not being able to work; that is, the patient experiences pain attempting those activities. Why do most people see a doctor? They go because they have pain. They do not go and say "Doctor, I bring with me an objective finding." Medical treatment is based upon problems with discs, muscles, and nerve roots, as seen on the MRI, in association with symptoms, such as pain on exam, and which are treated in various ways. This does not provide a basis to determine whether a patient can lift 10 pounds or 30 pounds. Clearly, the physician is in an inferior position to the physical therapist, who has props and exercise machines to evaluate the patient. Further, the physician sees the patient much less frequently than the therapist but is asked, "How much can the patient lift?" as a precondition to getting reimbursed for the visit along with the requirement for an extended description of the visit, all the results of examination, and the demand to provide objective bases for medical decisions that generally are subjective. If they were not subjective, you wouldn't need a physician; you could use a computer when the physician says that based on my experience and judgment this is what should happen, that opinion is disputed unless objective basis can be identified. After all this time is spent dealing with the paperwork, the physician is aware that the patient will expect an enormously detailed explanation and overflowing reassurances that the problem will go away, and that they will never have any more problems in the future. The physician is certainly aware that other patients who are not on disability are happier, out quicker with less criticism of the results of treatment, with fewer desperate emergency calls from the patient asking, "The insurance company says your note didn't justify any more disability and cut off my payments. Why did you tell them that?"

MEDICINE THAT TASTES BAD ENOUGH

The patient who is convinced that their problem is much worse than anybody else's does not want to sit in a back school and hear a lecture. That may be appropriate for other people but not for them! Yet patient education has been shown objectively to be helpful in patients who have back pain and work limitations. In the Volvo factory in Sweden, where working is not as crucial to economic status as in the United States, a back school was seen to return patients to work sooner. The back school provides anatomical information about what is causing the problem, first aid exercises for the pain and as therapy, and about how to lift and to sit as well as to pay attention to posture. Thus, the overall conclusion drawn is that education or greater information to the affected person is of benefit.

As a consequence, we see that the problem is not entirely a matter of having back pain, but includes the fear of being disabled. While some people write books, and some of those seem to hold out a cure for everyone, usually exercises or customary treatment, it almost seems clear that such books wouldn't be published if there were such simple solutions. Health professionals may solicit large numbers of patients with signs and advertising. Even some chiropractors have neon lights with slogans, such as Why Suffer With Back Pain as if they could cure all cases. If they could, I think the word would get out without advertising. Attorneys seem to fill the advertising spaces between the soap operas which prima facie, on the face of it, seems to imply an adverse effect on insurance costs—certainly, it is the patient's opinion that they will probably get the same settlement after the attorney's fee as they would without. But, in many cases, the system requires formality, from a legal sense, and the attorney becomes a necessary evil. While the timing of television advertising seems understandable, it is to target those who are not out working, the ads never stress that getting back to work through comprehensive treatment as their prime objective. In fact, total disability or failure to return to productivity benefits the attorney's percentage and probably is contributed to by the usual lack of eagerness on the part of physicians, or even avoidance for these particular patients—even before they have the attorney, but particularly thereafter. It certainly would be argued by many specialists in the area that it is in the patient's best interest to get back to doing something and everyone with experience has found obstacles to that goal from the attorney, who represents the patient's maximum benefit (and theirs proportionately), so they make an argument that maximum disability is their responsibility to represent the patient, whereas in human terms, maximum productivity benefits a human being in the long run.

This further demonstrates that there is a lot of information available in the literature about back pain and about comprehensive rehabilitation treatment that cannot be realistically transmitted to the patient in an office setting. Not only because reimbursement is declining, but particularly as specialty problems are treated by generalists, such detailed information is essentially impossible for the nonspecialist to keep up with. Further, the physician finds it increasingly difficult in a customarily busy schedule encumbered by paperwork and other concerns to add significant time for a specific patient's office visit with the educational components of the treatment. This is particularly true when a patient is concerned about the cost of the office visit, which may or may not be covered by insurance, and complicated by the fact that public impression of general practitioners, namely that they are not as qualified as a specialist or a spine surgeon, makes them unwilling even to listen to the information.

Without this information or particularly with the appearance of a conflict between the move-on-to-the-next-patient type explanation often offered by some other physician, the fear and anxiety associated with low back pain is worsened. I specifically recall a patient with whom I spent so much time that my office receptionist and nurse had interrupted me three or four times to remind me about the other patients and how far behind I was getting to try to get me to move on due to restlessness in the waiting room. I later heard from that patient who was charged the fee for a briefer exam than she had actually received, that she felt I had been too quick with her. The fact is she was not satisfied that I had addressed the problem, which was sciatica during her pregnancy. She couldn't be X-rayed and was likely to have significant improvement with delivery and relief of the stress of the weight of the fetus exacerbating lumbar lordosis after delivery. I mention this because of the evident frustration of a physician who is trying and accused of being short with a patient when it literally was not true; my staff timed it at forty-five minutes, and I billed for a twenty-minute visit. The frustration makes the physician wonder whether or not it is worth trying to treat these patients, when many other physicians refuse to see them, and particularly because they seem impossible to satisfy.

As a consequence of the lack of adequate communication of available information, there is, in addition to the fear and anxiety, a widespread feeling of desperation among many patients. This contributes to a fear of hopelessness among these patients who sometimes get to know each other and commiserate about their problem and the lack of effective treatment or relief, which acts to multiply the problem. Patients have had back pain that was attributed to disc problems in the last few years, but the same problems were thought caused by the sacroiliac around the turn of the century, and were either lumbago or rheumatism prior to that. The patients haven't changed, but vogue solutions seem to be most directed toward our concept of the problem that I will discuss in the next chapter. There is undeniably the generation of unorthodox solutions, perhaps second only to those given to cancer patients, that have caused back patients to give up on orthodox or organized medicine. They are well known for seeking in desperation any unorthodox solution that promises benefit. Certainly the information from medical sources is contradictory, confusing, and not well presented, and patients seem to feel that their complaints are not believed or heard. As such, the listening ear of alternative providers is eagerly sought as well as corsets, braces, magnets, exercise programs, special beds or chairs, and an enormous array of other telemarketed appliances.

We truly want to be guaranteed that our incomes will stay the same, we will have our current lifestyle maintained, our current pain-free status, and our plans for retirement. This guarantee may mean that we have to go through suffering such as having an operation, and if so, that's acceptable. It is not acceptable to have any interruption such as that caused by the problem of back pain! Hence, when we buy an appliance such as a washing machine, we are likely to be receptive to an extended warranty plan or some other form of insurance to minimize any possible disruption that a breakdown or the need for repair would have on us economically or otherwise. By analogy, we don't want to have a bad back interfere with our vacation, or with the promotion that our hard work has been leading toward, or certainly not to be at risk for recurrence down the road. The unpredictability of an episode of back pain, or the untimeliness of the disability, brings us back to the point that it is really fear of the unknown. As we learn more about the commonness and about the involved factors as well as the treatment, we should become better able to handle low back pain. As we recognize that nearly everyone has low back pain at some time, we have to understand that there are things that can be done for it. And, as with any other problem, if we can learn to deal with it, we will make it less fearsome by handling it, but certainly not by ignoring it. This book is intended to provide background information to the patient with back pain, particularly who has not been relieved by customary treatments so that with this information, the problem can be handled and literally put behind him. The next chapter will focus on the disease process or the pathology, which is commonly seen in patients with back pain.

EVERYTHING WORKS, BUT NOT COMPLETELY

One of the most difficult problems to deal with is the fact that low back pain may improve without being completely resolved over the customary arbitrary times allowed, say six weeks. It has been presumed that minor back problems should resolve after such a period of time and that failure to resolve is a consequence of the problem being more severe, hence surgery is often considered. Surgery involves the anatomic changes by a surgeon's instruments and techniques, for example, removal of disc material or bone spurs from pressing on a nerve. If there is pain but not disc material or a bone spur pressing on a nerve, surgery will add scar tissue to a problem and as may seem a little more clear later, is like the removal of an appendix for a patient with colitis, a technically perfect operation will not benefit this inflammatory and nonsurgical type problem. Surgeons evaluate patients by physical examination. Patients who have certain physical signs on examination as well as associated tests are selected as patients who are likely to benefit from surgical intervention. If these surgical indications are present, after other therapies have failed for a significant interval, then it is indicated and appropriate to proceed or at least recommend operating. Without becoming overly technical, many patients do not have surgical indications, but are frustrated because they are not better in a period of time which represents their limit of patience rather than the natural course of healing, or they have had previous episodes and they are sick and tired of these relapses and want to have it over with. As a consequence they may seek out a solution, like buying a new car not to deal with the repair problems. The reality is that surgeons do not give new car warranties or remake the spine, but rather provide specific anatomically describable changes to the spine to address specific problems that may or may not represent the entirety of the symptom complex.

The problem I perceive to be the most difficult is the patient who wants something done, who fears becoming a chronic low back pain patient and whose doctor has decided that nothing more can be done nonsurgically for the patient, who is dissatisfied with the results. That patient is then referred to a surgeon as an affirmation of the genuineness, and an acknowledgement that the doctor recognized how much pain there is. If this is an eager surgeon, operation may occur without careful analysis of the needed appropriate surgical indications. Unfortunately, without these indications, this patient is doomed to live with a poor result. The best situation is that the original problem remains, now with the addition of scar tissue. For the more careful surgeon, the suggestion is made to the patient that surgery is not needed. This patient then feels that the medication and exercises offered are not medicine tasting bad enough to be effective for the problem and hence conclude that the physician didn't believe or understand the severity of the problem, or that particular surgeon is not good enough to fix the problem. We will try to address this problem in the following chapters with discussion of causes and solutions with regard to low back pain.

It is my conviction that the surgeon who operates on the back is obligated by position to become familiar with methods of nonsurgical treatment and assure oneself and the patient that everything nonsurgical has been done before surgical intervention is recommended. Although this is not commonly the case, I think it represents an ideal for the best treatment of the patient and should be strongly recommended. The patient must have every opportunity to heal without surgery; not to quickly have an operation before spontaneous recovery eliminates the opportunity for surgical intervention. At the same time, the surgeon has a commensurate responsibility for familiarity with nonoperative care, and also a perspective of the true problem, which may be disability.

The person who is not a good candidate for surgery based on surgical indications will not return to work after an operation despite demands for surgery and assurance of intent to return to work, when motivated by severe frustration with results of nonoperative care. Unless the standard surgical indications are present, a good result, or relief of pain and return to function, cannot be anticipated. The surgeon must select patients who will benefit and must suggest to some that surgery may make them better, but not necessarily return them to work. In that case, light duty needs to be recommended from the beginning; and part of the problem is that the surgeon may not see that as part of one's purview or responsibility, although the patient presumes that the surgeon is not only captain of the ship, but the yeoman, pilot, navigator, steward, first officer, and deck hand. Although this is not realistic, the surgeon is in the public mind a higher authority in many cases and as such, the patient wants to hear directly the surgeon's opinion. Further, the insurance carrier seems bent on having a single treating physician or an attending from whom unified opinions and recommendations can be heard and not have to distinguish between conflicting medical reports. Understanding the inappropriateness of the insurance company making medical judgments, the surgeon is relied upon to give the most definitive opinion, which can then be used for insurance purposes. Unfortunately, the surgeon is best at specifying whether or not surgery is required and others, such as occupational medicine physicians, or physiatrists, are better suited to deal with issues of return to work; and unfortunately, the purposes of the insurance carrier are to minimize costs or exposure, which may not necessarily be in parallel with the needs of the patient for whom they are contracted to treat medically.

Failures of Treatment in Patients Who Have Back Pain and Become Disabled

Patients who have back pain and become disabled learn quickly that their insurance carrier is not a generous friend nor responsible for all of their problems that seem to result from this interruption in their working and subsequently earning capacity. From an economic standpoint this is understandable, and although they have an obligation from the liability which they undertook for premium received, if we are stressed by an illness and do not have cash resources to meet our needs, we understand; when it is someone's fault, then we expect them to pay for all the related factors. Not only do photograph developers limit their liability not to cover the cost of a repeat vacation if they destroy a customer's film, but travel agents are not responsible for the weather. After a short interval, it becomes clearer that the insurance carrier has a business interest in minimizing its expenses. This is not a handshake matter and their conscientious efforts to satisfy their shareholders will cause them to question reimbursements even that the patient will presume they must pay. The suffering and injured person will assert many claims in an effort to make his circumstances and life remain as normal as possible, expecting understanding and compassion, which is not a business concept. After the patient becomes frustrated with attempts to normalize his life and make provisions for family and economic needs, considerable hostility may arise against the insurance carrier, who in some cases seems to go to lengths that would strain the imagination to avoid paying for certain items.

Considerable discussion in the literature has revolved around depression, which is commonly seen in patients with chronic pain or chronic disability. This is certainly understandable, and caused by their inability to find relief for the pain or find treatment to allow resumption of normal activities. There certainly is also a problem with self-esteem, which grows and compounds as a person is unable to perform ordinary and customary tasks. The problem is that the patient who is unable to return to work becomes dissatisfied not only with the employer but also with the insurance company, often with the health-care provider, and then often with family and finally with oneself. The high incidence of family dysfunction and divorce which occurs during these periods certainly suggests that circumstances often create such a significant stress in these patients that they cause problems with the job that the physician is unable to address. Further, the patient needs to deal with issues, whether they are taking responsibility in overcoming obstacles, developing independence and not expecting assistance with every problem and this should be clear as we discuss active treatment as opposed to passive treatment in a subsequent chapter (Passivity).

The legal process is to make decisions, to adjudicate, not to truly remedy situations. Not only are there no winners, but after years and years of fighting, there is really no satisfactory solution for either party. When litigation becomes protracted, the delay leaves the patient irreparably a victim and the insurance company pays out not only the settlement and expenses, but legal fees in as well. While the judges who are personally unaffected may say that the wheels of justice grind slowly but they grind exceedingly fine, there can be no restoration of the lost time, the interrupted careers, the family hardships and agony from loss of income and opportunities that work injuries represent. Such is the case in, for example, Pennsylvania, where worker's compensation is excessively formal from a legal standpoint requiring every injured worker essentially to have a lawyer. This burdens the entire process not only in expense but with time delays, which are particularly damaging to the patient.

This is good for the attorneys; following the recognition and response to a similar problem in automobile insurance, we have no fault. This situation is not good for industry. In Pennsylvania insurance costs more to the employers, but the patient and the health-care providers are reimbursed less than adjacent states. Naturally these costs are straining our economic viability in this country, so it becomes a social problem as well as a medical problem. The purpose of the worker's compensation system was to protect the worker's income but any who have participated in the system are well aware that legal maneuvering often includes failing to pay benefits. Even if they are later restored, this forces the issue and is part of the legal system and maneuvering, which is customary, but violates the concept of income continuance, a basic tenet of the system. As the patient loses his car which was many payments behind, or even the house, the fact that this is later restored can never compensate for the bad credit, the deliberate denigration and the profit from maneuvering the legal system which is a legitimate exercise of right in the adversarial legal system of the insurance company. The fact is that patients cannot sue their employer for worker's compensation injuries; they are immune from that suit because they have agreed to pay continued income to the injured worker. Their children may lose opportunities in school, as well as self-esteem, when the parent's income is interrupted. Children may be unable to enjoy vacations and, after all, their childhood is short and ends. They may be in a very stressful family situation, leaving permanent scars from the temporary loss of income. They are denied some of those sought-after peer pressure clothes, or perhaps participation in a number of activities that their peers tell them how much they enjoyed. They are clearly innocent victims, due more to the system and the way it works than to the parent's injury. This situation is so common that most people can find an acquaintance, neighbor, friend, or perhaps even a relative or family member, who can relate to the difficulties and lack of satisfaction.

Many patients seem to fall between the ivory keys of this medical piano, considering themselves failures of nonoperative care, but who present to the surgeon without the appropriate indications, and thus are not able to get the operation, which they feel they need and are entitled. Unfortunately, they are really not given any hope. If some other avenue of nonsurgical care is recommended, they seem impatient having tried some other things and commit to having it fail, so they can have their operation. Even cancer patients are given hope. Perhaps in some cases there is a fear that back pain represents one of the classic warning signs from the American Cancer Society, as a wound that does not heal, a pain that does not go away, as an indication of a much more serious problem underlying, which their doctors have not taken seriously, believed, or bothered to investigate.

Real hope does not come from reassurances, such as all of us got from our mothers when we were young. All of our youthful anxieties seem to have been satisfactorily resolved as we grew up. Hope comes from being informed, feeling in control, and understanding what measures we can take to deal with a particular problem. The commonness of back pain would suggest that we should find it almost inevitable and survivable. Hopefully, an understanding of some of the conflicts between the patient, the treating physician, the insurance carrier, and between expectations of each of those will be addressed by this book and thus prepare people for problems with their back and give them hope that help is available.

The surgeon may understandably perform a less exhaustive search to find nonsurgical solutions than would be ideal, as a surgeon is in the business of doing surgery. In some cases it may be impossible for the surgeon to investigate the quality of prior treatments nor to repeat (under his own observation) the same conservative treatment, or be satisfied that all treatments done on the patient for many months previously and in some cases even for years, prior to the examination, have involved adequate nonoperative treatment a precondition to surgical intervention. Patients whom I see seem to have a strong desire to have physical therapy or other treatments near their home, as if physical therapy treatments are all the same. The convenient treatment is provided, but it is not certain that it is completely adequate. It is not under the control of the surgeon; it is not fully appreciated or evaluated by the surgeon to understand exactly what had been done. Suddenly, when the patient returns unimproved by physical therapy, the conclusion has been that surgery is needed despite my call as the umpire that they don't need surgery (or at least have a low likelihood of benefiting from an operation). This cannot lead to a satisfactory rapport. Any explanation that I provide will not satisfy the patient who wants to have it over with quickly so that he can go on with his life, get ahead, and have his back cut. Certainly patients who have been seen by a general surgeon and after evaluation are determined not to have appendicitis, such patients are not followed interminably by the abdominal surgeon for diarrhea or colitis or other abdominal matters, but they see a gastroenterologist.

As another example, when the primary care physician or internist refers a patient to the cardiologist, the patient can then expect either his cardiac medications to be manipulated for maximum medical benefit, or if there are specific indications or reasons, referral for a surgical solution. This solution may merge between the cardiologist and the cardiothoracic surgeon, in terms of invasive cardiology and percutaneous transluminal angioplasty, but the patient who does not have a large, juicy disc herniation is not going to have the dramatic benefit from a microsurgical discectomy that a patient would have if they did. A patient may have some benefit, but without the large disc herniation the benefit will not be as dramatic or the actual back pain can be worse from surgical treatment of the disc. As we will discuss later, the disc impingement on the nerve is more responsible for leg pain than back pain. The difficult matter is the back pain in some patients who do have disc disease. Not only do most all of us have disc disease when we get to be fifty, but one third of young patients with no symptoms whatsoever will have significant disc disease.

Many of these patients with symptoms of back pain, even with some leg pain, should not have an operation, not only because the disc is not protruding but more importantly, and this is usually totally unappreciated by the patient, their examination does not show signs of tension on the nerve from that disc pathology. As a result, their primary back pain will probably be unrelieved and any referred leg pain is likely not actually sciatica (radiating leg pain down past the knee by irritation of the sciatic nerve), so it won't be changed either by the operation. This may lead in some cases to the patient who is so eager to have the surgeon operate that the surgeon feels pressure to consider surgical intervention in a case where the disc herniation is present, but is neither large nor fails to clearly correlate on examination with a significant effect on that anatomically identified nearby nerve. Perhaps it is true that if this surgeon doesn't operate, another surgeon may, and in fact, the other surgeon may be less qualified, causes more scarring, and leave a worse result. Nonetheless, the patient who is told that his disc is on the wrong side and that he has right leg pain and a left-sided disc on the MRI often will very heatedly recommend to the surgeon, "Why don't you just take it out and see if that helps?" rather than understanding the meaning of an asymptomatic incidental finding. As such, the disc herniations may be unrelated to the problem even though they are generally accepted as traumatic and as a result of some accident or injury on the job; deterioration or arthritis may be present, with enough room in the spinal canal available for the disc to happily coexist with the nerve root and not cause any problems. This is not to say that there is not a problem, only that the disc is not the problem and, as such, surgery is not the solution. Further, the surgeon may not be the best person to find the nonsurgical solution!

Many patients are greatly distressed when they hear that they have a bulging disc and particularly when they may be told that discs are like tires and some of theirs are soft and one is blown out. Unfortunately, most of these patients do not hear from their doctor that there is no clear connection with how many gray hairs you have on your head and how bad a headache you may be having. I spoke at a meeting in a department store for active aging where I felt that the average age of my audience was about eighty-five years old. Following the talk, I was mobbed by these elderly white-haired ladies who told me that they had an MRI and their doctor told them that they had a bulging disc. I can surmise that they went to their doctor with pain complaints, the doctor was probably a general practitioner without specific interest or additional training in the spine, and felt obliged to explain the pain. Certainly, at their age, the risk of metastatic cancer or other problems was significant and investigations were necessarily performed, although the MRI may not be the most cost effective. Having had that study, to tell these patients that they had a disease was, in my mind, misleading. If they had a little deterioration in a knee or hip that was working fine, they would be told they had a little arthritis and would understand, but they were flocking around me because they knew I operate on backs and assumed that they may be potentially in need of my services, which was clearly not the case. As we will discuss in following chapters, their discs were so dried out that this bulging at their age was normal and the likelihood that they would herniate a disc was exceedingly low for people as they age, particularly past sixty.

Patients may delay calling and scheduling an appointment with the surgeon, presuming that surgery is eventually necessary. When no other hope is in sight and they have exhausted their resources and the resources of their family physician, they finally bring themselves to the point of going to the surgeon. At this point they are ready for an operation; but if the surgeon suggests that the disc is really bulging and not herniated, they can become indeed confused, disappointed, and may respond by getting another surgeon. The distinction between a herniated disc and bulging disc is, at least, open to interpretation. The severity of the problem, as emphasized by the pain, and particularly by the treating doctor or chiropractor with embellished explanations of the disastrous events that have occurred in the back, in an effort to encourage compliance with treatment and subsequent referral, may be hard to undo! As such, we need to remember that even if the disc is herniated, surgery is not necessarily indicated. As a corollary, we should suggest that not everyone needs to have an MRI. Perhaps everyone who buys a lottery ticket absolutely needs to have a color TV for the purpose of watching the televised drawing of the lottery, but it does not necessarily follow that every patient who has back pain, particularly those without leg pain, needs to have an MRI to see whether or not there is a disc herniation, as correlation with clinical symptoms is by definition already not present in the absence of leg pain.

A significant correlation with disability includes the fact that many patients who have meager education are involved with fairly heavy lifting or other manually demanding occupations. Such patients are really in a trap, and may have been told by their parents or their uncle or some family member that they should go back to school rather than go out immediately and get a job to pay for that new car that they can't live without. Thus, they have had some ominous self-fulfilling prophecies of doom from family members who have flagged or followed them in their eagerness to get employed. In particular, how many correspondence school courses, enterprises that are in your own home with meager venture capital and are part time, or other sales promotion gimmicks are sold to people who may be working in a manual labor position, but seem almost a form of disability insurance in their mind and have the intention of protecting the family if they are unable to support them with the labors of their back. Manual laborers certainly are familiar with associates and friends who have been unable to continue and will recite those examples to their children, who they suggest should go to college before getting a job, as their livelihood depends upon their health and the strength in their back. The disruption of income from an injury or a lifestyle from a back problem is widespread and well based, but again is an example of the fear that is commonly encountered, which I feel can at least partly be relieved by the available information presented in the following chapters. As Franklin Delanore Roosevelt said, "The only thing we have to fear is fear itself," and if we understand to a greater extent the problems that are a result of fear and not of the problem itself, the better we will be able to treat and analyze the problem objectively.

Insurance carriers seem to want to escape from the economic burden of injuries as opposed to illnesses that would be covered by other insurance. An advertisement in a travel magazine was prominently shown a few years ago where a young football player in uniform was on a stretcher, and that advertisement was intended to consider worker's compensation clients. The question was, "Was he actually hurt on the job or was it the result of an earlier injury?" I always found that ad confusing, since the laws are written to protect the worker's income and did not allow the insurance carrier a loophole in terms of a preexisting condition, which was then exacerbated. Clearly as the patient is working, the preexisting condition itself cannot be the cause of the disability, as their attendance at work on the day of the injury proves that they were not disabled from the preexisting condition. On the other hand, the low back problem that may have resulted from football in high school, which preexisted, could have been exacerbated by the proximate cause of the disability, that is, the new injury, and as a consequence the treatment and problem may be far worse than would be anticipated from the details of the accident and the extent of the actual injury in terms of physical forces applied to damage the spine. As a consequence, I have felt as a treating physician that this seems to be a fulfillment from the viewpoint of the larger picture, as consistent with the intent of the law to protect the worker's income. Unfortunately, insurance carriers are represented by adjusters or attorneys for individual cases, who often are unwilling to pay soon or without a struggle and this seems to worsen their costs. I take this ad, which was quite prominent for many months in several magazines, as evidence that the insurance carriers don't really understand that the law protects the worker's income in its intent, as explained to me by an attorney who, in 1916—1918 wrote for the law school of which he was an alumnus a textbook on the compensation law in its form at that time in the state of Pennsylvania. Certainly his qualified opinion of original intent differs greatly from the present impression on the part of many.

More importantly, the intent of the law was to reduce costs of litigation as well as delay going to court. I think it is hardly deniable that those goals have been circumvented in the present setting, particularly as strict adherence to rules of evidence and other procedural matters seem to require actual legal representation at each step of the process. Also, since the original intent was to prevent delay and legal expense by providing immediate and just compensation for wage replacement in return for the worker's willingness to forfeit the right to sue the employer, it seems glaringly evident that the entire process treats the worker as the accused and the physician as suspect. The treating physician is labeled nonobjective, attempts are made to favor the insurance doctor (versus the patient,) who is rendering an opinion favorable to the company, as if unaware of the Hippocratic Oath and the responsibility of a physician to a patient. Finally, the insurance company is the bad guy—in no decision or any proceedings that I have ever heard has the company been criticized or had consequences recommended for treatments that had been delayed even if in bad faith (the patient has to live, if not in suspended animation while the court decides). The literature shows that the greatest responsibility actually may lie with the employee's immediate supervisor. As physicians, we are familiar with patients who have recovered but refuse to return to their previous work environment (divorced people do remarry, but not usually each other). An angry boss who puts stress on the worker beyond his ability to cope, cannot be discovered or even noticed in the present compensation system.

Unfortunately, this is not like a fender which was damaged in a motor vehicle accident and can be repaired when the insurance issues are settled. Namely, the person is in the meantime unable to work, hence requiring replacement wages, and in pain, requiring treatment. If the employer would decide not to pay the claim and consider it not their liability, the patient needs to have something for the pain and the employee needs to cover his lost wage. The proverbial piece of straw that broke the camel's back leaves us with a difficult situation far out of proportion to the piece of straw. This preexisting condition of having a full load, not unlike rust in a damaged fender, certainly requires more than removing that last piece of straw from the camel's back. We all know that if you hit my car with yours, the bent fender may be banged out if it is new, but the rusted fender will probably require replacement when it is damaged by the collision, and that becomes your expense. The disability that threatens a patient's income may require expensive medical treatments and may involve underlying conditions that were, in fact, present at the time that the patient or litigant was working unimpaired but result in a much higher expense and more extensive treatment. The problem is not whether the referee decides in our favor, nor whether the insurance carrier is liable, or even whether the compensation payments are going to be continued to the worker. The real question is, as life goes on in any case, can we be truly objective and contribute to overcoming the anger that is generated in the worker about the situation that this person is involuntarily subjected to, and get that patient in the midst of litigation and in the midst of their pain, to look over the situation and say, "What is the best thing for me to do and for my future?" We must proceed on that basis, putting the backache behind us. The person who sees oneself as the victim is in a prison from which there is no escape. This is a purpose served by rehabilitation and the type of program often referred to as functional restoration, where the perspective is changed from "What can't I do?" to "What can I do?" and what would be the best plan to pursue for my future and for my family's benefit.

Chapter 3

PATHOLOGY

No man is a good physician who has never been sick.

—Arabian Saying

Pathology is probably an unfamiliar word, but simply means the study of disease. From a medical standpoint, laboratory procedures are performed by the department of pathology and include the analysis under the microscope of tissues from biopsies, blood tests, cultures (the examination of pathogens for infection), and also where autopsies are performed to better understand the disease process in cases that have already been fatal. Sufferers of low back pain need to realize that their problems are not all identical, that it is not always a disc rupture problem, and as such the treatments or results will not all be the same. Nonetheless, it probably will be disc related, that is, disc deterioration, which is identical whether it's due to aging or an injury, and probably is as inevitable as getting gray hairs on the head. By that same analogy, the graying of the hair is gradual, occurs at different ages in different individuals, pretty much always happens, and thus carries no grave concern; disc deterioration should similarly be considered common in different individuals of varying severities at different ages, and not by itself feared any more than the inevitable consequences of growing older. In this chapter, we will look at the various problems that are commonly seen to occur so that the reader will have a general understanding of the types of problems commonly encountered by patients who have pain in the back.

Disc Problems

The disc is an important and fascinating structure that has been studied extensively. It is known, for example, that the inner part of the disc, or the nucleus pulposus, contains interesting molecules that love water. Water is drawn in and held by these long chain molecules called proteoglycan (Figure 2). The ability of these proteins to draw in water is dependent upon their structure and, as we might expect, deteriorates with age. As proteoglycan is studied in older and older individuals, the chains are shorter and molecules of water are less avidly held, leading to a situation where the nucleus or center or the disc essentially desiccates or dries out with age. We know that normal aging results in the need for bifocals because of dehydration in the lens of the eye, making the lens too stiff to focus closely. We know that by a different mechanism the stiffness and water retaining (shock absorbing) abilities of the discs and other component parts of the spine also dehydrate and deteriorate as a result of aging.

It is interesting that astronauts actually gain height in the absence of gravity to squeeze the water out of their discs, which is drawn in either normally when we lie in bed or to a greater extent for them in the weightlessness of gravity . We are also aware that returning astronauts have back pain and must sit in recliners. This is partly because their blood vessels fail to maintain the muscular tone needed to support their blood pressure up to the head and brain. They are gradually reaccommodated to the influence of gravity by slowly progressing from a reclining or lying position toward the upright posture. In addition, the slow introduction of gravity allows the accumulated water to extrude gradually from the discs, back to the patient's circulation. The astronaut resumes customary height as well as relief of pain from increased disc pressure when returning to gravity. Fluids going in and out of the disc are absolutely essential since they are the only forms of nutrition to the tissues within the disc.

As water is drawn into the disc and disc's swelling causes a significant pressure, we appreciate the fact that this can be the cause of some pain. Clearly the astronauts have pain when the discs are full of water until time and gravity cause the water to squeeze out and equilibrate to a normal situation. But they also have considerable pain with an abrupt change. The

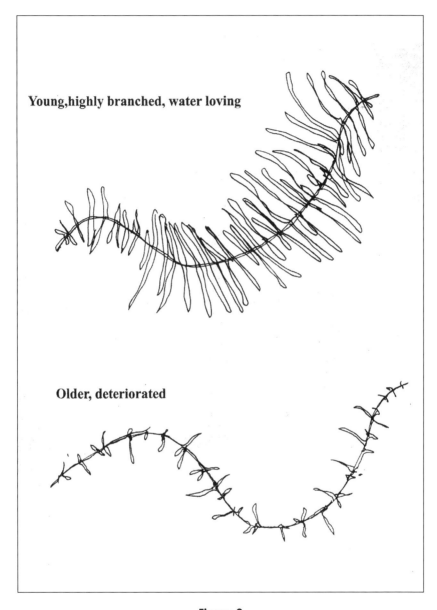

Figure 2

Long branched molecules of proteoglycan, particularly hyaluronic acid, tightly attract water molecules. The avidity decreases as they deteriorate and shorten. The upper molecule is younger and would be more hydrated than the lower, aged molecule.

pressure in the disc at some time in the past was considered to be one of the crucial factors in causing pain in the back. Patients with back pain were thought to have increased pressure in their discs and this was later thought to be a reflection of the bulging of the disc, although, bulging discs probably have no increase in pressure. Pressure measurements were performed by introducing transducers as needles into the discs of volunteer patients and the pressure inside the disc was compared in various positions. As a result of this, certain positions were thought to be dangerous and others were shown to be therapeutic. That is, the pressure in the disc is about equal to body weight when a person is standing and a smaller fraction of that when a person is lying. Hence bed rest is confirmed to be a valid treatment for a disc problem. Sitting, on the other hand, causes an increase in disc pressures to 1 1/2 times body weight and sitting in a chair and leaning forward to pick up something at the floor level can increase the pressure in the disc to more than twice normal. Hence, sitting is a stressful activity, which is confirmed by disc problems and spine problems generally experienced by truck drivers, from the vibration of the road, independent of and in addition to the stress of material handling, that is, loading and unloading. This is also time for salespeople or people who just do a lot of driving in their occupation. This information provides us with the perspective that a patient who complains if they have more pain sitting than they do standing may very well, if other factors also correspond, be complaining of pain from a disc injury or a deteriorating disc. This has to be remembered when we provide sedentary light duty for patients who have a back injury and then question their credibility when they still have pain just sitting and not doing any of their previous lifting or standing.

The study of the incidence or frequency with which diseases occur is called epidemiology. From that study, which has confirmed disc deterioration and injury from road vibration in truck drivers and salespeople, we also have documented a correlation that is evident with patients who smoke. Back pain is more severe and frequent in individuals who smoke, as well as their having more disability and more frequently required surgical intervention. By injecting a needle into the disc and measuring the oxygen tension within the disc, it has been learned that smoking causes deprivation of oxygen to the tissues of the disc by fifty percent; with three cigarettes a day this adverse situation is maintained. Hence we know that beyond poor nutrition, by inactivity, preventing the ingress and egress of fluids by motion, squeezing fluid in and out, as well as a lack of exercise or therapeutic motion, that smoking even a small amount causes severe oxygen deprivation to the cartilage tissues which otherwise would maintain the long chains of the proteoglycan, maintaining their water retaining capabilities. This is significantly interfering with the normal, healthy physiologic state. Further, smokers have a great deal more cough, including chronic and even productive coughs, and with such we would expect an increased pressure in the spine that is often associated with an exacerbation of sciatica or spinal pain or even disc rupture; though there are other mechanisms, clearly the strangulation of the tissues without oxygen is undesirable.

In fact, as the deterioration of disc material continues, we have a problem with clumping in the nucleus pulposus, the center of the disc, from deterioration or aging of the proteoglycan. The homogeneous uniform water absorbing nature of proteoglycan is altered and it mechanically clumps, like curdled milk. These clumps are between two flat surfaces of the end plates of the vertebral body. We can consider the analogy of a marble between two books; if we move the books, we would expect that the marble is soon going to be pushed out of the space between the two books. This situation suggests to the spine surgeon a mechanism for the common disc rupture: an asymmetric force, either rotation or side bending, such as commonly is seen on the job, when items to be picked up as part of your work are not situated always directly right in front of you, this becomes a typical story for many of their patients.

As deterioration progresses and as forces are applied, either repetitively during the course of a day, or with a sudden fall or other accident, the portion of the disc in the center which has clumped becomes a rupture. The rupture, if it presses on a nerve, may cause sciatica and sometimes may benefit from surgery. The ruptured disc or herniated nucleus pulposus which does not press on a nerve is likely to cause pain in the back and inflammation, but over the course of months to years, a disc will scar and stiffen, and will be tolerated with resumption of normal activities. Hence, we have the statistics earlier presented that ninety percent of people are better from the back problem within three months. However, there are a few percent who have continuing problems and benefit from a surgical procedure in which the portion of disc material offending the nerve and causing pain down the leg is removed. This operation is reliable for relief of leg pain, but is not directed at restoring the injured disc or relief of the back pain. In fact, one report has suggested that fifteen percent of patients after a disc operation will have greater back pain than before the operation.

Most persons are familiar with the concept of a disc problem, such as a slipped disc or ruptured disc, or generally an injury to one of the discs in the back. This problem is accepted as the result of specific trauma in many cases, particularly when an activity or accident at work precipitated the pain. As this pain is unrelieved by any measures following occurrence, it is then attributed as having been caused by that particular episode, but our scientific knowledge reveals that this is not likely to have occurred without previous clumping of the disc material or preexisting deterioration. This is not generally accepted by most individuals with a disc rupture because these are generally individuals in their thirties, although it extends up into the early forties and down into the late twenties. At this point these workers have not become familiar with the ravages of time; they are not arthritic; they are really in their prime of life and in a sense consider themselves still on warranty. When we consider the amount of force that is required in the laboratory to produce a disc herniation, we have such an enormous amount of force that it seems to exceed what would be expected in any activities of daily living including heavy work. When a disc is stressed above what is calculated to be the normal stresses of working on a repetitive basis eight hours per day we find that the disc is a very strong, hardy structure which does not fail. However, if we take the disc and make a defect in the disc such that it has a weak area, the amount of force which is required to cause a disc rupture or a herniation is within the level that might occur on the job, does not require the eight-hour-day repetitive stress and becomes something quite understandable. The weak point that we make in the disc which is used in the laboratory is not dissimilar to the natural history of aging or deterioration of the disc, which would be present and would make the disc vulnerable to a disc rupture at a relative low stress level.

When the surgeon removes a disc rupture, what is encountered at surgery is a fragment of fibrocartilage from the nucleus that found its way through the annulus and out into the canal where the nerves are and caused problems. This material is clumped up, grasped as a single piece, and represents a preexisting condition of degeneration of the nuclear or the inner disc material. Young patients who have had disc material removed for correction of spinal deformities, such as scoliosis, present with an entirely homogeneous and uniform material which you would expect to ooze out like toothpaste if the annulus or the donut containing the disc were injured. The material that is normal and is present in youth would not rupture and could not be plucked out by grasping the forceps, as is routinely done in surgery for a disc rupture. The clumped piece comes out as a single fragment. The young patient with a normal disc, who has a scoliosis being corrected, at surgery has disc material which cannot be removed by using forceps; you have to use instruments to spoon the material out. The clumping and deterioration of the inner disc or nuclear material are common in aging and the predecessor of the common disc rupture; in fact, clumping must precede a disc rupture. Deterioration occurs in terms of the water retaining capability as the disc scars or collagenizes to form these clumps, which then can be herniated as a result of some specific identified trauma or injury, for example, an auto accident or fall or even a twist of the back performing duties on the job. This deterioration becomes the result of an injury that is attributed to trauma, but is almost always preceded by molecular changes and a significant interval of time which actually occurs in all persons with aging, as we will contrast later to the simple deterioration of arthritis which occurs in the hip or the knee.

Since the scientific report by Mixter and Barr in 1934 connecting sciatica or leg pain with a rupture of material from the disc, as discussed in the historical review of Chapter I, attention to a large extent has been focused on the role of the disc in back pain problems. Although surgical techniques have improved through subsequent time, the procedure is similar in intent to that original operation of removing pressure from a nerve. Imaging studies have improved and have attempted to identify disc ruptures which would benefit from an operation. The surgeon uses these imaging studies as a road map to go to exactly the place where the disc material is located and then to remove any pressure from the nerve. The size and extent of herniated disc materials can also be estimated and this can give the relative degree of compression on the nerve root. The newest technique, the MRI, can show disc deterioration in patients who have no pain whatsoever and in fact, almost everyone. Further, at least a third of pain-free people have a bad disc and a majority of patients over fifty years old have significant abnormalities in their spine; however, these may be totally asymptomatic or they may be significant problems.

Pressure on the nerve results in loss of function of that nerve, either numbness or weakness. That is, if the nerve is a motor nerve as its function, then the muscles innervated will be weak or will fail to work. If the nerve is sensory, the area served by that nerve for sensation will have decreased sensation or be hypesthetic. Nerve pain is a matter of inflammation or irritation of the nerve, with or without compression. Clearly a lot of nerves have some level of compression and if you relieve the inflammation for example by an injection or by medication to decrease inflammation, the continued compression may cause that inflammation to return. Research has specifically investigated the lack of correspondence between the amount of compression and the amount of pain. It has been discovered that there is an inflammatory component which is the part of the back pain; however, there is also a substance P, which seems to be the factor significantly associated with present pain, and it is more important than the physical size of the disc material or herniation impinging and contacting a nerve root. This area has had continued study and research, hence a mechanism is further being studied for the generation of pain. It is not possible for an abnormal MRI to predict the benefit for an individual who has an operation, even though that surgery is successful and has been done several hundred thousand times a year with excellent results. Patients need to be evaluated by a skilled practitioner who knows their entire history, the events relating to their first having pain, and what makes it worse or better and so on, their physical examination, their imaging studies, and everything taken together to make a clinical or a subjective decision. We should be reminded of the fact that when we acquire a particularly shiny new hammer, we can have a lot of things look an awful lot like a nail. Owners of that new hammer might start swinging at some things that are not really nail-like and may not have the desired result. This surgery is not new (since 1934) in terms of modern medicine in which a new drug or techniques come out regularly and make major changes. As of the time that disc surgery started, we did not really have antibiotics or significant control over many of the infectious diseases that have been conquered in recent years; but from the standpoint of many surgical techniques, this could be considered relatively recent.

Surgical indications for the spine, and specifically for disc operations, are relatively straightforward: removing pressure from nerves can relieve neural compression. Unfortunately, the severity of the pain is not part of that criterion and some patients who have severe pain may not have significant neural compression and may not as a consequence be improved with surgery. Certainly there are other problems that cause pain, and there may be the need for surgery for instability or treatment for fractures and even extensive surgeries, but the concept that most people have in their mind is not consistent with surgery being for nerve compression. People seem to think, first, I had a terrible problem, I went to the doctor, he agreed with me how bad and how terrible was the problem. Because of the severity of the pain he decided that we had to operate; I could not be expected to live with this. The expectation is that the operation resulted in complete restoration of the spine to normal, no further pain or problems or limitations, and then I promptly returned to my workplace and all of my leisure activities as well. This does occur on many occasions with disc herniations and with a properly done disc operation, a microsurgical lumbar laminectomy, spectacular results can occur in the right person.

This occurs when it is: (a) the disc problem (b) that disc herniation is causing the pain and (c) there are no other problems. Surgical indications have to take into account the fact that asymptomatic patients, that is, no back pain whatsoever, may have a significant disc herniation on an MRI, CT scan, or even a myelogram. These patients should not be operated on because they have no pain or problem and they function normally without any restrictions. Nonetheless, if a patient comes with one problem such as back pain and has a CT scan done revealing an abnormality (in at least a third of normal people, and increasing as we get older, almost all MRI scans were abnormal when patients were in their sixties), the surgeon must carefully review that study, taken together with the clinical situation. The clinical situation, which is to correlate the findings on the MRI or the X ray with the actual physical examination of the patient. This includes palpation for tenderness and history to describe the location of the pain, as well as tests of either the reflexes or of provocation of the pain in a radiating manner (straight leg raising), and finally evaluation of the distribution of either numbness or weakness on manual motor testing. What this really means is that if we have pain down the leg, particularly to the foot or toes, and the leg pain is worse in the back, then this is an indication of a pinched nerve, probably by a disc. If the location and distribution correlate with the findings on an MRI, it would be "correlated", and that patient would be expected to have the good result from surgical intervention. The operation on a disc is not an operation which is expected to help back pain. Frustrated, angry, disabled, and genuinely in pain patients may want an operation, but it is predictable that surgery will not help them for back pain, and not unless they have specific neurologic signs and symptoms of pain in a pattern called sciatica will a disc operation be beneficial. The physical examination which includes the location of the pain and the reflexes, as well as provocation of the pain in a radicular manner (straight leg raising) and weakness on manual motor testing, is to correlate clinically that the finding on the MRI film is the cause of the pain.

This problem of a herniated nucleus pulposus, or a disc rupture, has to be on the same side as the pain and has to correspond neurologically with the nerve root involved in terms of the patient's symptoms, and should be large enough to appear to press on the nerves as seen on the imaging study to be the cause of the problem. In fact, there is a direct correlation between surgical result and the size of the herniation, bigger herniations giving the better result, or the harder you are hitting your head against the wall, the better it feels when you stop. Some large disc herniations have been treated without surgery successfully; and in the long run, that is, ten years later, according to a study done twenty years ago in Denmark, patients ten years after the disc rupture were the same, whether they had the operation or not. This does not negate the value of surgery, as patients were much better in the first year, and many dropped out of the nonsurgical group to have the operation. If we live in a socialized system where it doesn't make much difference in terms of our income and lifestyle whether or not we work for ten years, then we could accept the result more readily than under our current situation where a substantial difference in income and lifestyle is dependent upon whether or not we are able to work.

A patient who can return to work with only minor residual pain does not absolutely need any operation. This may go contrary to the desires of those patients who want to have their back restored to warranty standards and get it fixed since it's covered. If what I have presented is understood, a mild residual pain is not likely to be improved by surgery. A small disc rupture may have a small benefit, but we have a multitude of sources which may be causing the pain. In fact, there may be residual pain after surgery that is often attributed to scar, or may come from other sources than the disc, but also may come from the disc. That is, if a patient has instability, that would require stabilization of the disc or in some cases a fusion. Having back pain and not performing a fusion would be expected to fail to relieve the back pain as relieving pressure from nerves would be expected to relieve radicular or radiating pain only. So the actual type of surgery is crucial to address specific problems and removing pressure from nerves or decompression (which is either laminectomy or perhaps microdiscectomy) will relieve radiating leg pain but it will not address segmental instability, so patients with back pain will still have pain and often present with worse back pain after multiple laminectomies. Certain problems such as low back pain and segmental instability are not fixed by some procedures, although other surgeries may potentially address those issues. There are some mild residual pains which are from scarring in the nerve before the surgery or from the surgery, and these need to be endured(lived with) as further surgery may actually make the pain worse. Further, in special cases such as when the patient does not have preexisting loss of disc height, that is, that the disc is not bulging and deteriorated for an extended period allowing the bones of the vertebrae to come closer together than they were when the disc was healthy, then this particular patient may be a candidate for some of the more interesting new technology, either a percutaneous discectomy (Band-Aid surgery) or a laser discectomy. Both of these seek to remove material from the center of the disc allowing either some disc material to return into the center of the disc and away from the nerve, or at least to remove the pressure on the nerve. Although these procedures have a lower percentage of good results than the open operation, in the selected patient they can be performed and may be satisfactory. Patients who have a poor result may require the standard operation which, rather than being outpatient, will require hospitalization for a day or two if performed carefully. Although my preference is to include the operating microscope, results are excellent, either with magnification on the glasses of the operating surgeon (loupes) or with the operating microscope, so the major risk of the percutaneous or laser procedure is that the standard procedure may be required if the pressure on the nerve root is not adequately relieved by removal of disc material through this route.

Dissolving the disc or chymopapain had been introduced under the FDA and then withdrawn to be subsequently reintroduced, but has had diminishing popularity subsequently. This is mainly because nearly half of the patients have severe muscle spasm after the injection of the enzyme, which far exceeds the pain and discomfort of an open microsurgical procedure. If having a one-inch incision is far less painful for most patients than having an injection, and the results of the open procedure are superior to those of the injection, then it follows that even fear of having an operation is not sufficient motivation to risk the pain and discomfort that too commonly occurs with the enzyme digestion. Perhaps most of the percutaneous procedures are replacing the use of the enzyme so that rather than enzymatically dissolving the disc, the material is percutaneously removed either through suction or with laser dissolution into vapor. The problem is that the back pain and muscle spasm associated with the injection of the enzyme, which theoretically would avoid scarring around the nerves, would suggest that the material is not entirely contained within the disc. Thus, scar tissue will occur around the nerve roots and in fact is commonly seen as a problem in patients who have had papain and has to be a major consideration, as it is an irrevocable change with which many patients who have had chymopapain have to learn to live with for the rest of their life. One caveat should be noted: if a patient has enzyme or chymopapain and does not have a good result, that patient should have an open operation soon, as the scar tissue that is most commonly seen following a failed chymopapain is an irreparable situation that may be improved by early operation before the scar is established, allowing removal of any disc material that may be near the nerve root. Although it would be worse than the primary procedure, that is, without having previously done something, it is usually better than the result of waiting and seeing or, specifically, better than late operation which is commonly unsuccessful and disappointing. Unfortunately, it is difficult to propose an operation that soon after a procedure, technically an operation but felt to be an injection or the avoidance of surgery.

FACET SYNDROME

About the same time as the disc and its role in causing sciatica was being described, another phenomenon called the facet syndrome was described, in the late 1920s and 1930s, which is where the small joints, or the facets at each level were noted to have pathology. That is, they deteriorated or became arthritic and in elderly patients there may be spurs which press on nerves. This is a coupled response (Figure 3) from the disc drying out, losing height, and disrupting the alignment of the facet joints. In fact, studies for the Arthritis Foundation have shown that the injection of chymopapain to decrease disc height by dissolving part of the disc results in a predictable and repeatable experimental form of arthritis in the facet joints, which has been studied to learn more about arthritis. Besides the change in position, this causes the facet joints to no longer meet together with an exactly corresponding shape. That is, one side of the joint is intended to be facing its mirror image so that the two sides match exactly. When the alignment is changed by a loss of height in a dried-out disc, the facet joints no longer exactly match and thus some areas of the articular surface will have concentrations of stress, or even point contact, and will not wear evenly. In addition, the balance of weight distribution between the portion borne by the disc and the balance, which is borne by the facet joints, will be disrupted.

This could be called facet arthropathy, where the diseased facets have undergone a degenerative process which may or may not have a recognizable representation radiographically, or may not specifically have X ray changes until bone spurs develop, as this may occur quite late. This problem then becomes difficult to treat and diagnose because we do not have the ability to clearly image it in black and white to define the problem and then to evaluate treatments or results of treatments. Disc ruptures are seen well on MRI and CT scan, and arthritic spurs are seen well on CT scan. An

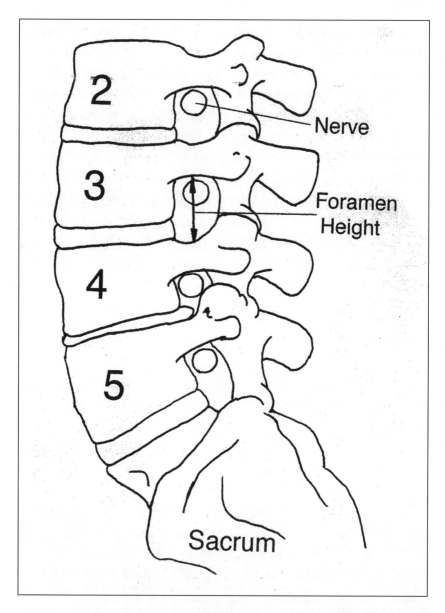

Figure 3

Each vertebra has a bony "body", which is separated from the adjacent vertebra by a disc. Loss of separation between the body of L4 and the body of L5 narrows the foramen correspondingly. The upper facet on L5 enlarges (spur on the superior articular facet) and may cause impingement on the nerve when bending backwards.

unsatisfactory facet joint, that may have deteriorated articular cartilage and may be causing pain, may be catching or locking and causing the patient to have severe pain with muscle spasm, such that they drop to their knees with the back "giving out", and which may be interfering with the patient's life and occupation, may occur without a characteristic appearance on our objective imaging studies. Hence, patients who have injuries to the facet joints often will have what is called in the legal field soft tissue injuries, and there is hence no objective finding to demonstrate for the patient that they are entitled to compensation wages, leading to the fact that a dispute results between the insurance carrier not wanting to pay and the patient with pain and no income replacement feeling that they are not believed. This is an area of active interest under the NIH perspectives and other research interests to see whether injecting these joints for relief or other avenues would be helpful to identify and evaluate this syndrome. Unfortunately, some patients who have facet joint problems and have substantial relief of their problem with injection have undergone a fusion procedure. To this point, those fusion procedures have not reliably restored the patient to full function, suggesting that it is a more complicated issue or perhaps that a facet fusion is inadequate stabilization or another procedure is necessary.

As we have briefly discussed, the natural history of the spine includes degeneration observed throughout recorded history and occurring in various forms. That is, the facet joints are part of the same bone as the vertebral body in front, and as the space between the vertebral bodies decreases as the disc loses height, the alignment of the facet joints in the back is altered. While this does not qualify for what we would customarily call medically a joint subluxation, the alignment is not exact and, of course, we are talking about two surfaces of a joint, so much like two links in a chain there is no fixed position for the links, as they are movable. Nonetheless, there seems to be an alteration, either in tension on the capsule surrounding the joint or relative position of the two joints, as well as in the in the relative proportion of weight bearing shared between the disc and the facet joints in the erect position, so that the situation is disturbed and has been widely studied but not exactly described. The result is that pain may be generated, and that exercise or manipulation may result in some relief, either by altering the position or by stretching out the surrounding soft tissue. At least some of the manipulations done by chiropractors and osteopaths result in an air explosion in the facet joints, the same as we would have by cracking our knuckles, and we could understand that the air explosion (cavitation) would give an air cushion for that joint to be loosened up to move more freely and to relieve the pain, but it would not result in a permanent change in the structure. As a consequence, if we rehabilitated the back in the meantime, that may lead to progress; however, if we go to the chiropractor passively to be manipulated every couple of weeks, the end result, after prolonged treatment, is nothing in addition to that passive modality.

The contrast with the patient who has a disc problem is that sitting causes increased stress on the disc; if the patient has a facet irritation, they will have more capacity to accommodate the nerves in the spinal canal when they are flexed forward as in the sitting position. Hence, relief is by sitting rather than worsening or exacerbating the pain in the low back. Further, they feel worse when standing, which provides a measure of relief to the patient with a facet problem unlike the problem of a diseased disc. The diseased disc and facet arthropathy go together, as it is a coupled system, but the mechanics are relatively straightforward. The facet joints are oriented in a vertical manner. As a consequence, one will slide on the other in a forward bending motion; however, when we both bend and twist, the joint surfaces impact together and precipitate problems. Generally a twisting injury or some combined movement from poor body mechanics or poor lifting techniques will precipitate the back giving out and an acute episode of pain and disability.

When the facet joint or, particularly, the capsule of the joint is damaged, either in a single episode of trauma or from repetitive over-use, the restraint, which the facet capsule would customarily provide is not maintained. As a result, stability falls back upon the need for muscle tone, which may be inadequate after an injury or repetitive stress to stabilize the spine. Hence, the individual feels, when bending a certain way, that the back gives out. As a consequence of this recurrent and unpredictable problem, much frustration occurs and the patient who feels unable to do necessary tasks when they are at risk of having their back give out, for example, when they work on a ladder or on dangerous platforms or at a height, they may feel they should have an operation to prevent this problem from occurring. Many of these patients do not have a disc pressing on the nerve, as they are fine prior to the giving out of their back, and hence they would not benefit from the anatomic change resulting from an operation on the disc, even if there happens to be an MRI finding of a disc herniation. That is, disc herniations are seen in people who have no pain just as there are gallstones seen in many people who do not need the gallbladder out. An incidental appendectomy may be done when you are taking out the gall bladder; "while you are there" you take out the appendix so it won't later be a problem. Unless the disc is herniated and causing a problem, you should not be there! If the examination does not provide correlation of the pain with the demonstrated disc herniation, surgery cannot be predicted to be helpful and should be avoided. In fact, as the discs lose height by deterioration and the vertebral bodies come closer together, this can increase the stress on the facet joints in the back and in fact may be worsened by having surgical removal of some disc material, leading to worse problems.

This situation of deterioration in the facets or early arthritis and the clinical symptoms which are encountered with that situation is probably the most common presenting problem. Although the late symptoms of arthritis may be absent, such as sclerosis of the bone on X ray and loss of space between the joints, the joint cartilage may be damaged (which is not yet seen on X ray) and there may be an effusion or swelling in the joint with increased fluid within the confines of the capsule of the joint. The problem that really follows is that the pain in the back is intermittent so it becomes hard to describe, is quite severe, but presents suddenly and often, maybe so transient and quickly relieved that we forget the exact details and find it hard to give a believable description. More significantly, the facets are not well imaged, so we do not have objective evidence to document the severity or the underlying location of the problem, yet the pain may go part of the way down the leg, not usually below the knee, and this presents to many patients and even to many physicians a great deal of confusion such that they are not able to distinguish this problem from true sciatica or nerve root irritation.

It is not hard to understand that the facet joints should deteriorate following loss of disc height or specific injury to the facet joints, and this seems reasonable considering the fact that everyone expects to have bifocals from drying out of the lens of their eyes, and natural processes result in drying out of the discs as well. Just as predictably as in the experimental model where loss of disc height will result in arthritis, it can be seen almost universally in elderly patients on autopsy; unfortunately, facet deterioration seems to be present even in young people who have died from other causes and are examined after death. When we have pain and we do not have on physical examination the findings that would suggest a disc herniation which would be an indication for surgery, we are left with the situation that gives low back pain its reputation. This is, a patient who is greatly troubled by a problem that won't go away, which interferes with important activities, which is disrupting the whole outlook on life, and which the doctor seems neither to understand nor to be able to help. This probably is most similar to the situation a hundred years ago in which physicians presenting to the doctor had a 50-50 chance of being better, as most of the medicines prescribed were cathartics and laxatives to get rid of the evil humors. Perhaps it was partly in reaction to this empiric nature of medicine at that time that Dr. Still developed osteopathy and Dr. Palmer popularized chiropractic in some forms that we would recognize today. It is probably because of the lack of medical progress, specifically in treating this problem, or more particularly in obtaining and disseminating information on this problem, that chiropractic remains so successful, popular, and prominent today. This is despite vicious attacks and resistance by the AMA, which has persisted as an unjustified lack of cooperation, or even hostility in some cases, as the legitimate goal is patient care, not the supremacy of science. My conviction is that many of the perceived cracks of the back are actually a manipulation of the facet joints, as already cited like cracking the knuckles, but current studies are investigating the internal disc derangement syndrome and may represent the possible shifting of nuclear material away from the nerve root, as we do surgically, from some forms of manipulation.

The best we can do for the facet syndrome is to recognize it and to understand the underlying natural aging process, which is either accelerated or advanced by trauma. Perhaps for this problem, either on the job or with other pursuits as we will describe later, our most effective treatment starts with exercise but then requires a comprehensive program to accommodate or work around a problem that we cannot cure but which we need clinical insight to recognize. Several studies have attempted to identify facet problems by relief of pain with injection of local anesthetic. Subsequent fusion has not predictably and reliably resulted in improvement in these patients and thus cannot be at the present time recommended. Thus, if there is a relative loss of stability between the disc and facet joints, we try to replace it by strengthening the muscles in the same sense in which we would replace stability of a damaged anterior cruciate ligament in the knee by strengthening the knee muscles. Similarly, the back muscles should be strengthened to restore stability and function. This becomes a significant problem when it is complicated, as was discussed, by the patient who is anxious to get back to work, but whose employer feels is not motivated and interested in coming back to work. Certainly the employer does not want the patient returning unable to do the job that they were previously hired for, and frequently complaining of recurrent pain just like the last time with seemingly trivial inciting episodes. That is, picking up a pencil and having the back give out is a common scenario for many patients, but not impressive to the boss who is standing nearby.

The worst problem is covered in detail in the next chapter, and that is the passive attitude, "Doc, just relieve the pain, and take care of the problem." We should then return to our analogy to sports medicine, that is, strengthening the knee will functionally replace in many cases a looseness or lack of complete normal tightness for some of the ligaments in the knee. While a great deal of controversy has been generated over whether the facet problem should appropriately be surgically fused or stabilized, most cases are not that severe, as many cases of anterior collateral ligament laxity are noted which do not require reconstruction. There are, however, increasing indications that degenerative joint disease occurs following anterior cruciate rupture and there seem to be a great many patients with back pain and symptoms that mimic this facet syndrom, who potentially with present technology could be satisfactorily fused and rehabilitated with essentially a savings by paying less for the surgery than is customarily paid for permanent lifelong total disability. The athlete who recovers in the common day treatments of considerable technology recovers solely based upon an absolute determination to perform the vigorous exercise program that is concomitant with in some cases surgery, and particularly because of that individual's commitment, not of a special role of the exercise machine other than as a means or tool for the injured athlete to use.

Unfortunately, in injury cases we have a different concept. If you back into my car and damage the bumper, I may not only expect you to fix it, but for your insurance carrier to cover my needs in terms of a rental car while it is being repaired. If I backed into some object and performed the same insult to the bumper, it might be acceptable for me to leave it as is. Back pain patients have this perspective, as the athlete cannot hold his competitor responsible for the accident that caused the injury, but the employer is held responsible by the employee, for example, for having failed to clean up the oil on the floor on which they slipped or for other causes of accidents. It is, however, the intent of the worker's compensation system to create a no-fault system; that is, wages are replaced as part of the bargain that includes the employee's inability to litigate against the employer who is indemnified by the system. It is unfortunate in this situation where the employee sometimes expects restoration without any shortcuts or even regard for the economics of what the insurance company may be forced to pay out, until they feel that they have been completely restored, which in fact may not be possible. Unfortunately, we are dealing with an injury which mimics natural aging. We are not dealing with a warranty, rather with employees who are hired on an as-is basis, which has to include the natural results of aging. Hopefully this perspective will help us understand the merits of the arguments on each side, not only the company and insurance carrier who need to get the job done to remain in business, but also on the part of the employee who is in pain and whose dispute may result in loss of income for an extended period while the employer is trying to become convinced that it is actually a result of injury rather than aging or natural causes.

SPINAL STENOSIS

The natural progression of the previously described facet joint dysfunction would be the progression of arthritic changes which occur on the facet joints as a result of the mismatch of the mirror image of these joints, and as a consequence, the eventual production of bone spurs. The arthritis changes result in increased stress on the joint and on the capsule (the structure going from one edge of one side of the joint to the other, and thus enclosing the lubricating fluid within the joint, or the synovial fluid, which provides nutrition to the joint's surface, like the boot over a ball joint). As a consequence of the wearing down of the cartilage or the slippery surface of the joints and the inappropriate alignment of the joints with the loss of height of the disc, there is increased traction on the capsule as the joint moves in normal and abnormal ways and subsequently becomes more mobile or lax. As a result there will be pain or inflammation at the insertion or attachment of the capsule onto the edge of each side of the joint and as this information persists, the bone edge where the capsule is being pulled will have calcium laid down, or the production of new bone. This new bone has been referred to by some as a calcium deposit, although it is not just a deposit of calcium as we would have in arteries with arteriosclerosis, but it is actually new bone that is being produced normally in an abnormal place and because it extends into the direction of the capsule and sticks out as a spur. This is the basic origin of the spur, and in joints where we have arthritic changes and these spurs are forming, the result is a stiffening or stabilization of the joint. We thus expect less flexibility as we have changes in alignment and have weather-related pain or other activity-incited arthritis pain as well as general inflammatory problems. Actually, most of these changes occur quite undetected by the affected individual and are noted as they progress to a significant extent in patients who are often sixty and older as a narrowing or spinal stenosis of the spinal canal.

The spinal canal has a certain amount of room that is predetermined for a particular individual and must accommodate the nerves that pass through and are protected by the bony structure. On the front side, we have the disc that can bulge or herniate back toward the nerves. On the sides, laterally, we have the facet joints which can have increased fluid or swelling, within the joint capsule, causing a local irritative phenomenon as well as some mass effect from swelling. In more advanced cases, as we would expect under this heading of spinal stenosis, bone spurs take up room and narrow the available space for the nerves within the spinal canal. In addition, as the vertebral bodies come closer together with loss of disc height, the ligamentum flavum buckles as an accordion gets larger when it is brought together and this presses in from behind or in back (posteriorly) in addition to the facet joints which are behind the nerves but actually out to the sides. As this progresses, we have a tightness that can impede the normal flow of nutrients and removal of metabolic by products and thus circulation can be impeded by increased pressure. The pressure can be acutely exacerbated by increased swelling, such as the day's activities (walking or working). This leads to the observation that patients walk and find that after a certain distance their legs start to hurt or become weak and numb and at that point they need to sit down. This has been called neurogenic claudication and is present in patients who have narrowing in their canal. On an anatomic basis, bending backward into extension is more likely to decrease the amount of space in the canal. Hence, the upright position is a problem when the swelling increases from any activity, however minor, and as the severity of the narrowing progresses, the nerves are pressed sooner until the patient sits down to relieve the problem. While sitting the spinal canal is opened, even though marginally, and this allows a temporary increase in swelling to be relieved and as the swelling diminishes, the nerves are no longer pressured and thus the patients can resume their activities after a brief pause.

Some cases involve nerve compression to the extent that the patient has difficulty not only walking, but significant pain down into the legs just standing or lying flat in bed to sleep, and as this becomes progressive and interferes with the person's activity, surgical intervention may be considered. The surgical intervention is actually removal primarily of the spur, that is, the part of the superior articular facet that has a spur on it and impinges on the nerve root. To illustrate that, the facet, as we have mentioned, is the mirror image of two joint halves which are the lower, or inferior, facet of the upper vertebra and the upper or superior facet of the lower vertebrae. That is, on Figure 3 the L4-5 facet joint has the inferior (lower) facet of L4 and the superior (upper) articular facet of L5. As we would see from the oblique (angled from the side) films, or especially on a good quality sagittal MRI but here for simplicity the side view illustrated in Figure 3, the superior articular facet may have a spur which comes up and impinges on the space available for the nerve root as it exits the spinal canal. The space is less and decreases with bending backward, bringing the spur up into the nerve.

The problem we commonly see is not only that there is a general narrowing in the canal such that there is back pain and weakness in the legs after extended walking, but specific motions of the back may result in the spur actually pinching the nerve and causing identifiable specific pain down the leg in the absence of any disc herniation. The pain is elicited by bending backward rather than forward because the pressure is exerted from the back side of the spinal column. Although we are not really certain whether the chicken or the egg comes first, disc deterioration is common as is facet joint irritation and these are coupled, so they both occur; however, it is probably true that in a majority of cases one or the other comes first—we do not know which! Deterioration of the disc is common and of the facet joints and usually this is troublesome for many individuals at the ages between thirty and fifty; spinal stenosis with identifiable spurs usually occurs later in patients who are sixty years of age and over. The problem that is more common for the younger patient who has had a recurrent troubling back problem after an isolated injury or industrial trauma is that they may have a damaged facet joint or a damaged disc with associated facet joint spur which subsequently follows this injury and deteriorates at a rate far accelerated beyond the age at which their other joints have progressed and deteriorated. Although this is a process identical with aging, and some patients may have aging that appears in a sense ahead of their years, an isolated severe spur following an injury would logically be the result of damage that occurred in that area. On the other hand, it cannot be conclusively said that natural aging wouldn't start someplace, as some people may develop a shock of white hair on one part of their head and not white hairs evenly distributed throughout the whole skull. We do see in relatively younger people who have particular risk factors as we have described (vibration from driving, such as with salespeople, truck drivers, and forklift operators, and twisting and bending as is commonly seen on an industrial production line or factory work, and so forth), we do see generalized spinal stenosis, but we also see patterns that are limited to a couple of specific levels.

As we have discussed, the deterioration of facet joints is not shown well on any of the imaging studied, but MRI does show disc deterioration and the MRI or CT scan will show spurs, if the process has proceeded to that point. Injection of the facet joints or around the nerves (epidural injections) may be helpful to document the level at which the problem originates and are often done by pain clinics. The objection that seems to be unresolved is whether these injections are truly helpful or only temporary. That these injections are of only temporary benefit is certainly the impression of many patients and has support from the literature, particularly for a herniated nucleus pulposus, that is, a disc, as opposed to spinal stenosis, where we have arthritic elements similar to changes in arthritic knees, which are routinely injected. Although many physicians view the injections as diagnostic to identify and confirm the problem with a potential for postponing or delaying surgery, even if inevitable to a more elective basis, there are also sympathetically mediated pain syndromes that are dramatically affected by epidural injections. These are often referred to pain clinics in an effort to have pain management services, but instead they may only get injection services and the comprehensive perspective is lacking. The literature has supported comprehensive management, but specific resuts of less than comprehensive duplications have compromised results when they are not truly comprehensive in their rehabilitation techniques and facilities. Certainly there has to be some consideration for inflammation from a specific fall or accident which may be resolved by an injection, but the recurrence after a period of a few months would suggest that the joint is now irreparably damaged and surgical intervention may be necessary.

Any motion in the spine which seems to cause these recurrent problems or results in the back giving out can be obliterated surgically by a successful fusion. Unfortunately, other parts of the spine depend upon motion for nutrition. For example, the disc fusion locally at one level does not eliminate all motion nor does it guarantee relief from all residual pain. Obviously, if we expect to have a dramatic result from surgery, we need to identify the problem exactly prior to surgery and perhaps relieving it with an injection would be most diagnostic or convincing. Further, a fusion requires a significant time for healing, as opposed to a disc excision where we are looking at a convalescence of roughly a year as opposed to a few weeks. So, identification of the problem by a selective injection again seems reasonable before we embark on such a long therapeutic path. Nonetheless, several studies have been done of patients who are identified by injection to have facet problems and after facet fusion or spinal arthrodesis, they did not have the kind of successful relief of pain that would not only be expected but which should result to justify this significant operation. Indications for a fusion remain controversial and technical and beyond the scope of our discussion here.

This end result of aging or disc deterioration and facet arthritis results in spinal stenosis which occurs in the retired or elderly population, particularly those on Medicare, being treated as a disease. That is, if it interferes with their normal activities to an excessive extent, then surgery can relieve the problem and will result not in a new warranty or return to factory conditions, but the ability to do expected activities of the patient's age, a result considered reasonable. The problem is that we have many patients who are in their fifties and have perhaps worked many years at a particular job who may even consider themselves still on factory warrant; and as they have quite a few years left before retirement, they economically need to continue to work, but may have a recurrent troubling back problem. The surgical solution is improvement, not a cure, and certainly it is not unreasonable to expect that the results will not be the same as for a disc patient in their thirties. Nonetheless, the company has a job which this patient was performing and they may refuse to provide light duty or any accommodations. In this sense, we need to recognize the limitations of surgery as not curative or fully restorative as a result of deterioration, which preceded, although it did happen on the job. As a result, this deterioration may be considered a result of years of working; but if it is viewed as arthritis, some would interpret that as bad luck, not a compensable injury. Thus there is no objective result to be expected, nor a predictable outcome of the compensation case.

In these patients, we may selectively help some with surgery, if our expectations are moderated by their experience and age. As with early arthritis in other joints, such as the hip or knee, we prefer that patients be older and have less physical activity as a result of their age before artificial joint surgery is entertained. In the interim, before patients have gotten to be sixty-five and would be expected to do well with a total joint replacement, early arthritis is best tolerated. If we live with it and don't expect a completely pain-free result, then rehabilitation is the course we should follow, and perhaps I have partly gone through this entire explanation for the goal of convincing the reader that it is in their best interest in many instances to live with the problem rather than expect resolution, even with surgery.

FIBROMYALGIA

In some patients, we have a condition which has in recent years been preferred to be called fibromyalgia, although ten years ago the preferred terminology was fibrositis and has been variably called fibromyalgia, fibromyositis, myofibrositis, or muscular arthritis. All of these conditions refer to an inflammation or a subjective feeling of the muscles being in knots, which cannot be confirmed by any specific pathologic disease or changes in the microscopic appearance of muscles if they were to be biopsied and thus examined. The American Rheumatologic Association has progressively described and delineated this condition, which may occur as a disease, and as a generalized over-the-whole-body problem. It is also recognized that this problem may occur in a localized area after an injury. This is distinctly different from the common muscle pull. A backache may result from injuries to the soft tissues and in many cases this would be attributed to a muscle that is torn, swollen, or injured in some way. These backaches will generally resolve promptly with little or no treatment and would not be expected to result in that person buying this book. As a consequence, we are then restricting our discussion to those who fail to respond after an arbitrary period such as six weeks, when the soft tissues of the muscle or whatever illustrative reference is made to something that is injured would have healed. The insurance carriers would like to declare that soft tissue injuries automatically, uniformly and in every case, particularly the ones that they are responsible to pay for the medical costs and wages, do heal and there is no further claim after an interval such as the arbitrary six-week period. Six weeks would be forty-two days, Hippocrates said that sciatica was better in forty days; however, backache was not to be treated because it did not get better. Sounds like things are pretty much the same. Although some have stated an opinion that all soft tissue injuries are basically resolved in six weeks and after that any residual disability is not the result of the accident. We clearly appreciate a rotator cuff tear as a situation that sometimes requires surgery as well as an anterior cruciate ligament rupture. These soft tissues do not heal after any interval of time and this is the motivation for surgical intervention. Unfortunately, this is not the observed case as treating physicians have patients who continue to have problems; and despite the lack of objective basis, do not recover after any arbitrary period, and in fact, some may be permanent.

The concept of a soft tissue injury that does not promptly resolve, does not have objective demonstration on testing, and continues to interfere completely with the patient's ability to return to work, is not only a difficult problem but one the insurance carriers have been reluctant to accept as a diagnosis representing an injury. In many of the chronic cases and particularly where fellow workers do not find the complaints credible, some doctors evaluating these patients, rather than treating, cannot document any objective impairment or provide the physical information as expected and required of them for which the disability decision (a legal one, not the doctor's responsibility) ensues unfavorable to the patient. This is not to be critical of the insurance carriers, but is really a reflection of the diversity of opinions and the conflicting information they have to deal with. Naturally they prefer opinions favorable to their business. Nonetheless, patients who have a problem in which the muscles feel like they are in knots and are stiff do not benefit from surgery, feel improved with exercises and medication, but are seldom cured. This condition is particularly exacerbated by stress or tension in muscles. It is a condition that may be brought on by trauma, did not cause any problems in the past, may now cause intolerable pain, and be disabling after some injury which, in and of itself, has caused no X ray changes or herniated discs, and no demonstrable objective findings.

A similar situation has been described as a result of sleep deprivation. That is, if volunteers are prevented from entering into rapid eye movement (REM) sleep, then they will have sore muscles all over their body as a result of not resting. It is also observed that sleeplessness or a sleep disorder is commonly associated with this condition. This association has led to the search for a chemical or hormonal imbalance and underlies selection of some medication for treatment. It is clear that patients who have a lot of tension involved with their jobs are particularly prone to the continuance of the fibromyalgia syndrome. It is further evident that the deprivation in oxygen from smoking makes recovery exceedingly difficult if not impossible.

Further, these seem to be related as the addiction to nicotine is associated strongly with the behavioral component and patients in need of a cigarette will usually suggest that they need to calm their nerves with a smoke. Nonetheless, the tightness from increased tension and stress which manifests itself after prolonged periods is pain in muscles, and this may be an intractable situation after an injury causes an otherwise benign stretch or muscle pull.

Patients often emphasize emphatically that the pain is so bad that they can't get to sleep. Anxiety produces sleeplessness or an inability to cope either with circumstances or (particularly with) the boss, and this is not related to the severity of muscle spasm or pain. Organic back problems that represent physical maladies are generally mechanical in nature; that is, they hurt more with more activity, such as working, and these problems are almost uniformly comfortable in bed, not interfering with sleep. Patients who have had surgery and have severe postoperative pain always fall asleep, but these patients claim that they have 24-hour constant pain, which in itself lacks some credibility, and seems an exaggeration for the effect of seeking a dramatic treatment. There is a quote from 1926 that: "exaggeration is as common as malingering is rare," and I think that is very telling, as patients sincerely try to present the severity of the problem and try to be believable. They have a tendency to elaborate or even exaggerate, but in most cases I find patients entirely credible; only in an extreme minority are there issues of true ability to return to work with overt deception and mistruth.

We are reminded of the philosophy of the Greeks that the mind and body were both to be exercised and maintained in good health. Certainly physically fit individuals have fewer aches and pains, and if they do have physical problems, their recovery is enhanced by their good physical condition. Certainly patients who work hard or exercise strenuously will be relaxed following the competition and will sleep restfully. Soft tissues are most significantly involved in the conditioning process. The joints and bones may over the long term increase or reinforce conditioning, but short of joint or bone failure their function is unchanged. The muscles and soft tissues can be stretched or strengthened with exercise and specifically can lose their muscle tone actually in a matter of days from inactivity. Although we have not specified in an anatomic sense which tissues we are actually discussing, when we exercise and increase our state of well being, increase the blood flow to our lungs and heart and muscles by exercise, the mysterious soft tissues are certainly the beneficiary of this appropriate activity.

Fitness has become a more prominent concern as more people have become involved in recreation and have seen and experienced the sense of well being and health that is imbued by such programs. My experience has been that athletic trainers are often more effective than physical therapists in benefiting the patient suffering from chronic low back pain, not only because they are interested more in a gradual process of conditioning than the concept of recovery from an injury, but also because generally they seem to be more hands-on in their approach. Clearly, the best way to relax tense muscles is first to tighten them and then after that, to allow them to relax. This is understood by anyone who has been exposed to Lamaze techniques. A widespread awareness of the need first to tense muscles to achieve good relaxation has been accomplished through these programs. Beyond tensing muscles is the need to exercise them, to apply deep heat as we might in therapy, but intrinsically with actual blood flow into the muscles by use. This is not only physiologic and natural and holistic, but also extremely effective. It is not only effective, it may be the only way to treat fibrositis effectively; that is, to ignore the pain, to work hard, and to then enjoy relaxation of the muscles by a good day's hard work. It certainly is easy for the physician to say, "Relax." The tension associated with the job may be inescapable; and it truly is not the tension, but rather the way the employee handles the tension, not the stimulus but the stimulus reaction, which is responsible for the result. Job dysfunction or decompensation is a prominent and common predecessor to many industrial injuries or reports of conditions that have grown to a level of disability, although they may or may not previously have been present. From a medical standpoint, patients who have fibromyalgia may be helped more effectively than those who from an occupational injury standpoint have the additional stresses of litigation or controversy with their worker's compensation case on top of their physical problem. Certainly concerns about chronic fatigue syndrome may overlap fibrositis to some extent or have a similar patient constitution or overall health condition, but fibrositis is significantly worsened by tension. These patients commonly are cured with physical therapy or other treatments and then return to their job place to have an incapacitating recurrence when the stress of the job is again experienced. The comprehensive rehabilitative approach would seek to rehabilitate and help individuals work through simulated stressful job conditions to allow return to productivity and personal self-esteem and satisfaction.

SEGMENTAL INSTABILITY

While statistics are on the side of the majority, there are some patients whose discs do not scar, stiffen, and effectively stabilize the back for a sufficiently functional and comfortable result or for tolerable pain. For them, the resumption of normal activities and occupation does not occur. Some of these patients have been theorized to have abnormal motion occurring in the spinal segment, that is, between vertebral bodies where the disc is located, and this is called segmental instability. The criteria for what exactly constitutes segmental instability is subject to question and many spine surgeons are trying to identify exactly how much motion in the lumbar spine is acceptable and how much, when present, would justify the need for an operation to stabilize (fuse) the back. It may well be that an acceptable cutoff point of motion beyond which the spine is unstable may never be identified and that belief has been adopted by many. The problem that we have again is that many people have a lot of motion and no pain and some patients have a lot of pain and no abnormal motion or less motion than the patients without pain. This is reminiscent of the fact that a lot of patients (up to one-third) have a disc herniation on MRI without pain, and thus we have to again rely upon the physician's correlation between the examination and the X rays to make sure we are not treating the X rays rather than the patient.

Having decided on the basis of physical exam, background, and X rays and imaging studies that the patient either has traumatically induced segmental instability or may have a bony defect known as spondylolisthesis (Figure 4), the physician has to decide whether or not the pain arises from what is noted on the X rays and exam. Spondylolisthesis itself may be present in up to five percent of the population; and, of course, in most cases it is not a problem but only noted incidentally when X rays are done for another reason. When the physician decides that from clinical examination and evaluation the bony defect or the segmental instability is the patient's pain generator, that is, the disc is incompetent from a structural standpoint and responsible for the pain or the bony defect allows excessive motion causing pain, the treatment which would be recommended is to repair the bone defect or to eliminate the motion in the unstable disc by stabilizing the spine. Actually, results are well established for spondylolisthesis, in which severe pain has been noted with a natural history of progression and lack of relief that is interrupted by the performance of an operation. Segmental stability is difficult to identify and, hence, the natural history cannot be established when you cannot clearly isolate the cases. The operation that is done is called a fusion or an arthrodesis. As illustrated in Figure 5, bone is laid along the sides of the spine and allowed to heal itself to the transverse processes and lateral masses (facet joints) of the spinal column in the same sense as the fragments of a broken leg would knit together and heal. When these bone fragments all become one, that is, the bone that is present heals to the bone taken from a bone graft donor site such as the iliac crest (a part of the pelvis), motion is eliminated and pain may be relieved. There may still be scarring and there may still be minor pain, but that is, to simplify the description, what we had to do. This fusion procedure was recommended as part of the report of the first disc operation in the 1930s, but has not become a uniformly accepted practice or proven to be beneficial despite the elapsed time.

The problem we then have is that a patient with sciatica and a herniated nucleus pulposus, or a slipped disc, will after a routine operation be better in days and back to work in weeks. A patient who needs a fusion will be better in months and may be be back to work before the first year, but certainly not on the same time scale as a disc problem. In addition, several studies have shown that patients who had surgery for a disc with or without a fusion did not benefit from the additional surgery represented by the fusion. As a result, we have to return to the premise that if a fusion does not necessarily return the patient to full duty, then why not consider light duty without surgery? A successful fusion has in recent years been shown to be helpful in returning some patients to heavy duty. New techniques including spinal instrumentation facilitate and enhance the fusion's rate of suc-

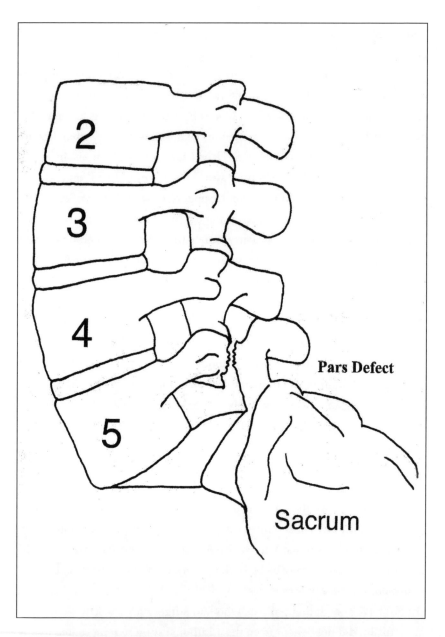

Figure 4

Spondylolisthesis is the forward slip of a vertebral body below allowed by a defect in the pars, or the part between the joints (pars interarticularis).

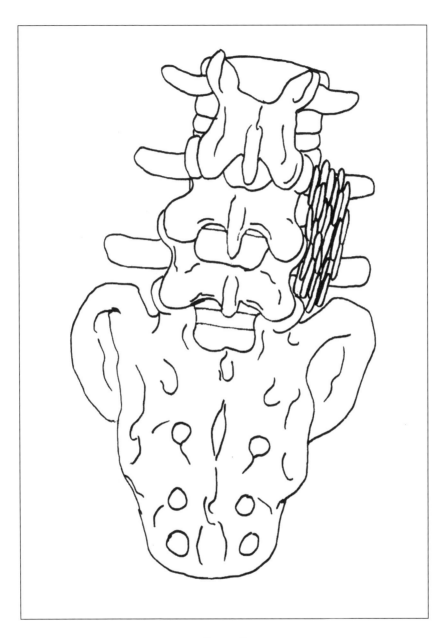

Figure 5

The intertransverse fusion or lateral fusion is by harvesting "match sticks" of cortical cancellous bone from the iliac crest and laying it on the paired in tertransverse process to heal into a solid mass of bone.

cess. The problem remains in selecting the patients who will do well having a spine fusion procedure; and many surgeons are trying to identify more carefully the indications that will result not only in the satisfactory operation from a technical standpoint, (for example X rays show solid bone fusion,) but also to determine the patients in whom an improved lifestyle will result not only by relief of pain but by increase in function and restoration of lifestyle.

Patients who have spondylolisthesis have a developmental problem where an area of bone has not formed. Some call this a congenital problem, but just after birth much of the vertebral column is cartilage and has not yet become bone; rather, it is during the first decade when cartilage transforms into bone, an area may remain cartilage without becoming solid bone in certain individuals. Unfortunately, the vertebral body is prevented from moving forward. One facet joint of the upper vertebral body contacts the facet joint of the lower vertebral body from behind prevents forward movement. When the part between the facet joints (or the articulations which is called the pars interarticularis or the part between the articulations) does not ossify, then it is possible for the weight of the body and other loads to cause that vertebra to move forward. As a result, these patients have a "slip" which involves displacement of the disc, the vertebral body moves forward upon the lower vertebral body, usually the lowest lumbar vertebrae on the sacrum. This is not a slip of the disc, but a sliding forward of the vertebral body, one on the other. Clearly in the absence of bone, fibrous tissues maintain stability or prevent the vertebral body from pulling forward. The problem is that these fibrous tissues may have pain fibers in them, which the bone does not, and thus the stress of the body may load those fibrous tissues and cause the pain fibers to fire a pain signal back to the brain. Causing a bony fusion will eliminate that pain and reliably relieve this problem.

Selecting patients for fusions is more often based (1) on failed previous procedures, that is, disc operations which produced temporary benefit but subsequently deteriorated, and (2) on patients whose X rays show that the spine has translation or moves forward slightly. In the spondylolisthesis, the "slip" may be greater when the patient bends forward than it is when bending backward or in standing compared with sitting. If the spine is then "wobbling," we have to consider it unstable, although as mentioned above, we don't have a threshold above which it is unstable and below which it is still stable. Basically, since the vertebrae don't remain in the same alignment, we consider this as the cause of pain. In other words, when the bony elements are deficient such as in spondylolisthesis, then rather than having bone to hold the upper vertebra from slipping forward on the lower one, we must have soft tissues which may have pain fibers in them. When we stand on our bones, we do not have pain unless there is a disease in the bones. If we have an area where bone is supposed to hold one vertebra back from sliding forth on the other but that bone is not present, then the stress of the weight of the trunk, head, and upper lumbar area will be imposed on soft tissues which may have pain fibers. If these soft tissues are firm, then we should have the normal situation where, in most cases, spondylolisthesis is noted as an incidental or unimportant finding on X rays. When, however, some of those firm soft tissues are torn such as in an accident or when an increase in the forward slip is noted on sequential X rays done at later times, then we would consider this to be a change, and if associated with pain, clinically responsible for the pain and thus a good indication to perform a spine fusion. If deterioration by loss of disc height results in some motion without the bony deficiency of the spondylolisthesis, we have a degenerative spondylolisthesis which may have similar results in terms of back pain and, thus, some of these patients may require stabilization or fusion.

This operation is a major undertaking as we have discussed. The patient has to wait for bone to heal and this takes a long time. Bracing is used as a trial to predict success but is a poor trial and limited in its effect. A sufficiently restrictive brace could efficiently limit motion of the spinal segments and relieve the back pain, and would require a force to immobilize bony segments in the spine that is transmitted through the skin. This magnitude of force may cause intolerable pain or perhaps skin breakdown, and that pain may exceed the pain of the primary problem. Pain from excessive bracing has to be balanced between effectiveness and being overly restrictive. The fusion has to be viewed as a last resort after bracing has shown that stabilization seems to help and an extensive physical therapy program causes muscle strengthening and stabilization. If the patient is clearly motivated in the physical therapy program and subsequently is willing to undergo a rigorous follow-up therapy program following surgery, the surgery is not likely to be curative completely , particularly as the patient will be immobilized from the swelling and pain for several weeks to months after and sometimes in a brace for an extended period.The healing of those tissues will require rehabilitation which, as the anterior cruciate ligament reconstruction in sports medicine, will require patient participation in an active sense.

OSTEOPOROSIS

Osteoporosis has for a long time been underappreciated, undertreated, and almost ignored. This disease is a major problem, the number one metabolic bone disease in the world. Diabetes mellitus really means that the urine tastes sweet and historically we are aware that physicians did not have the technology that is presently available. Despite excellent technology, however, it does seem at times a matter bordering on neglect to lack the availability of testing and technology for such a significant disease. Elderly women often have a senile kyphosis where fractures in the thoracic spine have cumulatively resulted in their thoracic spine losing significant height and being significantly flexed forward. It needs to be emphasized that this is truly a disease process and in fact may be preventable.

The balance of calcium taken in on a dietary basis and of calcium lost is, unfortunately, generally negative; most of us are in negative calcium balance from a peak density of calcium in early adulthood between twenty-five and thirty-five years of age. This situation develops over many years and the accumulated loss of calcium becomes severe with fracture risk encountered in old age. The problem that we have is that by the time this has occurred to its full extent, it is so massive a loss of bone that it is really too late to do much at that point. We can surgically treat hip fractures but the osteoporosis would be far better treated by some preventative and prophylactic measures in early adult life than to have to deal with the painful complications later.

Women have a higher rate of bone loss and start with less calcium at their peak bone mass. During reproductive years they lose calcium; but the problem gets worse after menopause when there is a highly accelerated rate of bone loss, and this continues for several years until the drastic increase in bone loss returns to the normal, somewhat slower, negative calcium balance. This is not customarily an occupation problem. It occurs in mature years of retirement and can be disabling. But more seriously, a significant portion of women after a hip fracture do not reacquire their full level of independence that existed prior to the fracture.

Osteoporosis is defined as a decreased quantity of normal bone. This differentiates it from an adequate quantity of bone that is diseased or weak. Rickets in childhood was formerly seen with a deficiency of vitamin D but that is rare in these days of food vitamin supplementation. More commonly we currently see metabolic errors of metabolism, otherwise rare but more common today than simple vitamin D deficiency; and in these cases the bone is soft, not properly calcified, or without the rigidity necessary for its structural purposes. In adults, the lack of vitamin D which effects the strengthening of bone and calcification of actual growth plates to achieve normal adult height may occur for various reasons. In adults who have already achieved full growth it is not rickets, but osteomalacia. Adults who have a decreased quantity of mineralized bone usually have other diseases that are at risk of causing these problems and, specifically, renal insufficiency or kidney disease where kidney failure, particularly in pre-renal transplant patients, interferes with the processing of vitamin D; and although all these patients may survive in our present area of modern technology, they do have complications from their diseases that take less priority than survival but have severe consequences for the patients that are so involved.

Understanding that osteoporosis is an inadequate quantity of normal bone, we then need to understand that bone is constantly being renewed and exchanged in the body during life. When this occurs after the completion of growth, there is a quantity of calcium and other minerals stored in the bones which is far greater than the amount of calcium that is available within the circulation for its various purposes. For example, muscles require calcium to contract, including the heart muscle; and many other enzymes or bodily metabolic functions require calcium. These functions take precedence such that the storage of calcium, which has been accumulating during growth and development, will be sacrificed if inadequate calcium is taken in on a dietary basis. Unfortunately, it is common that essentially all people are in a negative calcium balance; that is, they are in the process of losing stored calcium in their skeleton from a peak during early adulthood through old age. This situation can be lessened by appropriate dietary intake of calcium, particularly green leafy vegetables as well as milk, cheese, and dairy products and the consumption of a normal amount of vitamin D, which will ensure absorption in the gut of the diet's calcium. Unfortunately, the diet is generally not sufficient without supplements during pregnancy, or particularly for women after the loss of estrogen either through menopause or surgical menopause (hysterectomy with ovaries removed) to adequately lessen the process and prevent an actual disease process of severe loss of minerals and weakening of the bones.

The disease occurs in men, but just to a lesser extent than in women when calcium loss is accelerated by the reduction in the hormone estrogen at menopause, either naturally or surgically. Since women statistically live longer and start with a significantly lower quantity of calcium, they achieve a level of bone mineral density below the fracture risk threshold much more often than men do. Unfortunately, this occurs without any other disease; that is, it occurs in normal women. Women who have had certain diseases would be expected to have problems with dietary intake and the metabolism or the body's functional use of vitamin D and calcium, but this problem of osteoporosis occurs without any other abnormalities.

Manifestations of osteoporosis are the late findings and are often thought to be fractures particularly causing back pain. There may be fractures without back pain and these are incidentally noted on X rays and commonly seen. Unfortunately, they are usually seen along with fractures of the vertebral column, which do cause pain; and in the x-raying of those patients, other healed fractures are noted. Fortunately, these are what would be called stable; that is, they do not need surgical stabilization with rods and other equipment used for traumatic fracture, as they heal almost always without paralysis or affecting the adjacent nearby nerves when given sufficient time. During the acute injury or early time after the fracture, even bed rest may be required which then can be graduated to walking with a brace and finally to a resumption of customary activities.

In addition to the spine fractures, there are other fractures, principally of the shoulder or the proximal humerus, the wrist or distal radius, and of the proximal femur. These bones, even though osteoporotic, heal normally and in the same time as other adults, as a local priority of calcium need is established in some way by the fracture, such that the entire rest of the skeleton will contribute to accomplish healing in this area. It is a good idea to take vitamin D and drink milk after a fracture for the rest of the body, but it does not accelerate the healing, even in the severely osteoporotic patient.

Treatment is relatively straightforward, but not entirely satisfactory. We are able to lessen the loss of calcium but not reverse it until recently(with Fosamax), and research continues along this line. The general principles are to take calcium in adequate amounts, which would be generally 1.5 grams of calcium a day after menopause, or five dairy equivalents. Each dairy equivalent would be a glass of milk, a portion of cottage cheese or yogurt, or a green leafy vegetable salad. In addition, any daily multivitamin should provide 400 international units of vitamin D that would provide adequate calcium absorption by assuming normal vitamin D function of the gut. The fact that the damage from loss of calcium accumulates over a lifetime without any symptoms until it is really too late and the majority of calcium has been lost makes this an insidious disease. In addition to encouragement of calcium intake earlier, preferably in the thirties for most women, it has been shown not only that fractures are less common in patients who have calcium supplementation, but also calcium is lost less avidly by patients when they exercise. Whether it is the muscle contraction and increased blood flow and vitality to the bone or whether it is the stress on the bone which results in improved bone strength and mineral density, exercise is the most essential component when possible. Vitamin D is not really a vitamin in the sense that it is necessary in the diet—as with sunlight it is a hormone made by the body through the processing of cholesterol in the skin. Nevertheless, the intake of calcium without drinking an excessive amount of milk which would cause overweight problems, requires calcium supplements and it is appropriate to take a multivitamin to make sure that it is absorbed.

In much of the discussion of treatment, there is the mention of weight-bearing exercises. Women who perform normal exercises, that contract muscles and stress bones of the spine, should have far less development of osteoporosis over their lifetime, particularly, as they age. If they attempt to

keep active, starting in their thirties, then in the years following child bearing and child rearing it is possible for the calcium to be better absorbed and
potentially for osteoporosis to be prevented. While exercises will be discussed later and, particularly, extension exercises as well as flexion exercises, moving the spine backward as well as forward, the primary exercise and
the simplest is walking. Daily walking is good for weight control, overall
aerobic, or air breathing, exercises to condition the heart and lungs; and it
helps to preserve bone mass.

There are many new drugs that are currently being examined and are
reported to have promising effects; but the most significant is probably hormonal replacement, and it has been suggested that for at least seven years
after the natural onset of menopause, estrogen supplements should be
taken. This contradicts previous teaching, which was a concern that estrogen would increase the incidence of breast cancer. Actually, this has been
reversed and the incidence of breast cancer seems to be less in patients sup-
plemented with estrogen. Since a constant steady loss of calcium throughout life in men and women is present but greatly accelerated for the first
seven years after menopause, after which it generally reverts to the same
previously low rate, it seems protective during these years to take estrogen
to prevent that severe acceleration- a magnification of almost tenfold- and
the equivalent of another fifty to seventy years of calcium losses, leading to
such a severe deficiency at the end of this period that we commonly see the
fracture of the hip or the spine fracture or the other associated fractures.
Generally, women have little back pain unless there is a fracture, but after
fractures have occurred, there may be microscopic fractures in many bones
causing pain, which is best prevented by exercise, and common-sense recommendations such as avoiding hard-soled shoes and their impact on the
spine. New drugs are being developed and may dramatically improve this
disease but as yet we can reduce the symptoms and reduce the fractures by
about one half with vitamin D, calcium, estrogen, and exercise. The other
medications will require time so that we can present long-term follow-up to
demonstrate that they have not only helped but they continue to help after
an initial good start.

There are some drugs that been have made available which are bisphosphonates and these medications have been shown to help with osteo-

porosis. Conceptually, these might be understood in terms of a bank account. Osteoporosis is the imbalance of bone formation and bone removal, the normal metabolic action of the body to make new bone and to take away old bone. If we think of the body as having a skeleton that is a bank of calcium, then we take in calcium and make deposits; the body takes away old bone, making withdrawals. If we make too many withdrawals and fail to make deposits, we are going to be overdrawn and that is what osteoporosis is, essentially insufficient funds when the currency is calcium and the strength of bones to resist fractures. We may have minor areas of cracks in the bones on a frequent basis all over the body and these are repaired without our awareness. Unfortunately, major bones may break in old age as a result of severe osteoporosis and this is where we run into trouble. The bisphosphonates reduce the withdrawals. As the body metabolically turns over bone, the removal of bone is slowed by the bisphosphonate drugs. The newest of these is Fosamax which is probably in many women's magazines and of wide public awareness and is actually the first to be able to increase the density of bone. This is encouraging but has one remaining significant drawback. Fosamax is very poorly absorbed and as a consequence must be taken early in the morning before any food is eaten and only with water as even coffee or tea will prevent its full absorption. Further, the patient must remain upright because it has been reported to have an erosive effect about the lower esophagus. Nonetheless, this is the first drug that we have had which can actually reverse the process and increase bone mass. Further research should lead to new drugs that will be better absorbed, but for the present this is a significant improvement over what has been available. Optimistically, in the future better-absorbed medications will become available and this disease will be less of a problem from awareness, exercise and vitamin D as a prevention or prophylaxis.

MISCELLANEOUS

We have attempted to describe the most common forms of disease in the back, but certainly there are others. When a patient has pain at night, that is, without activity, then we have to be concerned about a process that is not activity driven, such as cancer or an infection. These are urgent considerations and, specifically, the symptoms of having increased pain at night which is different from night pain, the usual result of arthritis; that is, the accumulation of a day's activity results in pain at night as well as stiffness in the morning. But, when pain actually awakens a person already soundly asleep (which arthritis usually does not), then we have a situation that requires medical examination, at least X ray evaluation, to rule out these problems. As mentioned, night pain is also a sign of stress rather than necessarily being a malignancy or infection; and, thus, after a prompt evaluation to rule out other diagnoses, some appropriate response for stress has to be provided since resolution of swelling or healing of torn muscles or even surgical removal of a disc will not correct problems that may originate from the stress.

In addition to the inflammatory condition fibrositis, there are diseases from a rheumatologic standpoint such as ankylosing spondylitis that may also be present. Usually, a fuzzy appearance of the sacroiliac joints, a history of the problems with the gastrointestinal tract, or squaring off of the L5 vertebral body will be noted in association with ankylosing spondylitis or spondylitities. Of course, a major fall or motor vehicle accident may result in a fracture, and this should be self evident. Patients in an industrial situation may experience sufficient force to cause a fracture, and in some cases spondylolisthesis will be viewed as a fracture, although it may have preexisted in terms of a bone defect. Nonetheless, fractures, when present, represent a specialized case and will not be dealt with in detail here. Interestingly, we may mention that it is often the case that patients who are paralyzed from a fractured spine will find productive employment, accepting the fact that something is injured or damaged or different, but perhaps to some extent, the difficulties resulting in a large number of patients with back pain, without even demonstrable X ray changes or any findings other than dehydration or drying out of discs, often are totally incapacitated and unable to find not only the ability to work but any satisfaction or self-esteem for the remainder of their lives. This suggests that there is an element of fear that is an important component of the disability problem. Patients fear paralysis from the numbness or pain that they are feeling and they may be disabled by the fear that if they do anything it will progress; whereas patients who are actually paralyzed need to accept their impairment and proceed to resume any activities they are able to perform without fear and, thus, are not disabled.

We have not in this section discussed sacroiliac joints because they are below the spine, but they do cause backache and will be discussed particularly in the chapter on pregnancy, as the opening of the birth canal severely stresses the sacroiliac joint and that is a significant problem. This backache is associated with child bearing and even following childbearing for many months and, in some cases, years. Less frequent conditions are associated but these are beyond the scope of this discussion. Nonetheless, we have tried to present the major problems and provide some background information so that the reader can better understand that there are a lot of different types of problems and with that understanding also recognize that the treatments need to differ. They should be evident from the examples that many people try treatments and commonly are unimproved despite the fact that these treatments can be effective for large numbers of people. The simple truth is that if they have a different disease, different treatment is needed.

Hopefully, the discussion of what the actual problems in the spine are and how they are encountered will help readers to understand, as they are specifically interested in what their individual unique problem is and how it may fit into the overall picture, how their treatment is determined and how it fits into the overall scheme of spinal care and spinal rehabilitation. Having discussed the disease process as it is encountered, we will next discuss how the patient should view his role in the rehabilitation process by analogy to sports medicine and modern treatment for athletic injuries.

Chapter 4

PASSIVITY

For I believe that much of a man's character will be found betoken
in the backbone. I would rather feel your spine than your skull,
whoever you are. A thin joist of a spine never yet upheld a full
and noble soul. I rejoice in my spine, as in the firm audacious staff
of that flag which I fling half out to the world.

— *Moby Dick*

For centuries, it has been taught that we should respect the superior knowledge of professionals such as physicians and lawyers and should follow their instructions as being in our best interest. I recall this was a common theme on many "Perry Mason" episodes where the client failed to tell the attorney everything, vastly complicating and compromising the case. Certainly we are also familiar with information that we would consider patient education: for example, the fact that salt intake can influence our blood pressure. Further, we know that we must take our antihypertension medication or we will have the risk of complications like stroke or heart attack from high blood pressure. Finally, concentrated sweets can have a marked effect on diabetics who have to watch their diets. The prescription and therapeutic recommendations of a physician often depend upon whether the patient is compliant; do they actually follow the instructions or have there been some dietary indiscretions of either salts or concentrated sweets, or some other situation? Beyond the issues of whether we do what we are supposed to, the physician is also taught to ask questions about things that we are not supposed to do: do we smoke; do we admit to sexual activity which is unsafe, do we admit to excessive alcohol consumption and do we trust the medical system in the present age of computers to keep confidential information from being spread against our will? This is specifically an issue with HIV and psychiatric information, which seems to be more commonly a part of many patients' background medical information. Finally, we understand that failing to fully inform your physician of your compliance, noncompliance, or other practices can adversely affect your health. This is because the physician is taking care of you!

While patients may not be aware of a blood pressure higher than normal and may develop complications such as a stroke or a heart attack, they, therefore, are diagnosed as hypertensive and given dietary restrictions or medication by their physicians. They are to take the pills that their doctor prescribes, regularly and as directed, for the best result and for their optimum health. This situation is well understood, and much of our concern in medicine is not only the complexities of diagnosis or specific treatments, but matters of presenting that information in ways that will assure better patient compliance and understanding by education in the disease state and its treatment.

It is true for a disease model that the patient is passive and is cared for by the physician. In recent years, however, we have talked more about prevention and fitness, or health. Clearly, our well-being is promoted by losing weight, getting regular exercise, and being careful in our selection of foods and beverages. While losing weight is sometimes a medical issue involving medication or even surgery, it is by and large a self-enforced, dietary restriction program whose results depend solely on the participant, for even the dietician's help is ineffective without active participation. The exercise program that we undergo is solely a matter of our interest and persistence in doing it and actually putting out the effort and time to increase our lung capacity, increase our cardiac reserve, and strengthen our muscles. In these matters we are becoming increasingly aware of the role of the patient in taking charge and becoming actively involved.

Medicine teaches a passive attitude for patients, and even the position of the physician standing over the bedside of a patient established a dependency role that is diminishing in our society. Patients demand certain rights and they have expectations of the physician with regard to information and participation in decisions. It is a result of these changes and of our attention going to preventative medicine and good health that a commensurate responsibility is endued upon the patient; namely, that if the patient is making the decisions, the patient is also responsible for carrying out the actions, which may require substantial contribution in effort, time, and persistence. Government actions have viewed physicians as health-care providers or merchants. Thus, their product has to include consumer information. For the surgeon, this is coupled with a technical skill, but the end result and the coordination of the various components of service provided ultimately fall upon the patient as well.

Although it does not have to be emphasized to many persons that an active role is to their benefit, it is also outside of the awareness of others that their passive role is to their detriment and it may not be possible to make this point by the physician's instruction, or by the best physical therapist, unless a comprehensive program of rehabilitation or functional restoration is offered to those patients who need it.

Many patients present to the doctor with the complaint that their back "popped." This problem of the back popping has its analogy in the knee popping which usually represents a rupture of the anterior cruciate ligament. It is, however, likely that the cracking that is heard in the spine, perhaps more in the cervical but quite commonly in the lumbar, is similar to the knuckles cracking in the hands and should not be considered significant unless the popping sound is associated with pain. The patient may have, after several days, a pain that seems unrelated or perhaps a distant swelling that has occurred as a result of a torn ligament. Reporting to the doctor that the back popped leaves a dilemma, since ruptured ligaments are not likely to be revealed on X ray studies and many sounds can occur in the back without significant injury or change. There is, on many occasions, grinding that often is heard in the cervical spine because of the proximity to the ear, and that may represent degenerative changes in the joints, irregularities in the surfaces that result in noise like sandpaper rubbing on sandpaper, as discussed in the previous chapter. It is interesting that in many cases if a pop were heard in the arm or leg, many patients would go about their activities and see whether it interfered in any way. When something similar happens in the spine, there is enough emotional overlay and fear of chronic low back pain or disability that their action involves far greater concern and anxiety. In perspective, muscular tears are common and, as with muscular tears elsewhere in the body, usually these should heal within six weeks.

Nonetheless, if the patient has been at work and has a frustration level just about to the brim, is having difficulty coping with their circumstances, perhaps in some cases aggravated by other home situations or financial distresses of our modern society, and then on top of everything else the back goes pop, this certainly is a good opportunity to go to the first aid station or to the company nurse just to have it checked out. Whether cause or effect, the soothing of medical treatment may be welcome at a time of maximum frustration, or the lack of response on the part of the company nurse may in itself be the straw that breaks the camel's back.

Treating patients with back pain leads to many observations of patterns of behavior that seem similar from patient to patient. One of these is, "Please relieve the pain." This seems like such a simple request that the patient, often the spouse, and sometimes other family members, is overwhelmed by the failure of usually several physicians to relieve the pain. Why in this modern age of medicine can't we just relieve the pain? Physicians often respond by prescribing medication and then are distressed when the patient says, "That didn't help." This may even include narcotic medications. The real problem is that the pain is not a physical finding, but it is an experience. A back is not like a bent fender that you can pick up in three weeks after the body shop repairman is finished. If your back hurts and you lie down, you may find relief from this common medical treatment. However, if your back does not hurt and you lie down, in time you will have an aching back from being in bed too long. If you fall down and hurt your wrist, the immediate response is not to hold it absolutely still, motionless until you see the doctor, but to move it and say, "Well, that doesn't seem very bad. It's probably not broken." And if in a few days it resumes painless function; you don't even care to see the doctor. In fact, when some patients go to the doctor and have an X ray or go to the emergency room for evaluation, the real question is, "Will it get better?"

The same may be true for an ankle sprain. If it swells and seems to be severe, we present for an X ray, but if it is not fractured, we expect it will resolve in time. The same with the spine, but we don't treat it the same. If an ankle is placed in a cast for six months, at the end of that period the ankle will be stiff, motionless, and every time we try to move it, it will hurt. Yet patients seem to be under the same impression and, in fact, sometimes physician instruction, that they should lie in bed whenever their back hurts, as if pain in the back represents ongoing injury that should be heeded by absolute rest and immobilization. We expect, if we are not walking, that when we resume walking after a cold or illness that puts us in bed for two or three days, we will not be back to full function in all ways immediately, but we have to exercise and get back in condition. It seems evident that the muscles in the back would respond identically with any other muscles. If we have a sprain of those muscles, we should expect pain first, which may increase as swelling increases over a couple of days; then we should feel later that the pain is starting to resolve; but as it does, stiffness is left and the stiffness is lessened over time. We would not expect the pain to be totally relieved until some time later after we have returned to full function and are using those back muscles in our daily routine with more aching and soreness than usual, but not enough to alarm us.

When the wrist doesn't respond after a few days, we then become concerned that perhaps it may need medical treatment and we present to the doctor. When the X rays are fine, we are reassured and say, "Oh, that's great." When the back X rays are not fine, we are distressed, "Oh, no! Nothing can be done for me?" The passive comment, "just relieve the pain" is really the problem. The pain that the patient has is not the doctor's problem; it is not hypertension that would cause a stroke. It is a symptom and it is not something the doctor can fix if the patient is passive. Relief of the pain requires the resumption of normal activity, including exercise such as physical therapy in which the patient must be actively involved. If our wrist feels better and we are able to use it to pound a hammer or to use a shovel, but it still hurts, then we assume that in time it will get better; although, we may not be willing to return to work and all the other associated stresses and demands of getting jobs done on time and keeping up with our fellow employees and our expectations in terms of our performance that may be less than we generally achieve without evident impairment. That is, back pain is not visible. Some patients may feel that in the presence of their unresolved legal question or other stresses (as to whether they should be compensated for the time they were off, the job stress of what they may consider an unreasonable employer who is looking for an opportunity to terminate them or to fire them), their delay to work is (to them) an insurance policy that they will be able to perform at a level that they can continue in that occupation and not lose their job. When this situation arises, it may not only be a delay, but it may never happen that we are able to go back to work with the confidence that we can do the job or even be able when current treatment overemphasizes inactivity. Becoming actively involved may mean that we feel like we are working for the boss when we are at physical therapy and he is not paying us full rate, and it may lead to some resentment that they really should not have had that wet slippery floor where we were walking. It is clearly the case that any patient who becomes a chronic disabled low back pain patient suffers, and none that I have experienced would prefer their situation to their preinjury state; they consider themselves to have sustained a great loss. Nonetheless, they are trapped and many times told not to do things when resumption of those things may hurt only a small amount more than they hurt without doing anything, and might, in fact, be helpful in resolving the problem that is limiting their activities, their life, their ambitions, and their hope for future success and satisfaction.

Unfortunately, some patients seem to feel that medication and exercises are treatments that don't taste bad enough to be effective for them and, hence, they want stronger treatments. In many cases this is surgery or, particularly, stronger medication. Actor Richard Burton was known for his use of alcohol; but biographical information has suggested that back and neck pain, both on his part as well as Elizabeth Taylor's, and more prominently with former First Lady Betty Ford, who has been before Congress and in the media promoting treatment for alcoholism, dates to their use of prescription drugs for back and neck pain. The problem we see occurring is impossible to pin down or to quantify. That is, when is it necessary, or at least merciful, to provide some pain relief with an habituating medication or a narcotic for a short interval? And when is it being abused by the patient seeking escape from a pain that is really the expression of their inability to cope with circumstances, which in the usual setting is job stress. The fact of the matter is that narcotics are drugs which, when taken over a long period of time, have a diminishing effectiveness. There is, hence, a natural tendency for those medications to become less effective and to be demanded in higher doses. By the nature of habituation or addiction to narcotic medications, it is, therefore, contraindicated that these drugs be used on a chronic long-term basis. We anticipate that a patient who has diabetes will use insulin for the rest of his or her life. Patients who have arthritis anticipate using arthritis medication for the remainder of their lives. Patients with hypertension expect to restrict their salt, diet, and perhaps use medication for the entirety of their lives. Patients with pain cannot use narcotics and gain relief for any extended period, particularly not for the remainder of their lives.

In many cases, people with pain do not have an obvious anatomic site or a straightforward remedy, which can then be surgically or medically treated to eliminate the problem. Another problem is primary or secondary psychological factors and depression that become an accompanying component to this problem when it exists for a prolonged period. When the problem becomes chronic, it is often the case that the patients are unable to cope with pain, albeit they will be citing the many years that they have pain as a demonstration that they personally are of great intestinal fortitude and makeup, such that they have a high tolerance for pain: at the same time, they are describing the pain in terms or in actual words that suggest emotional or psychological components. That is, when patients frequently say it's like a knife twelve inches long stabbing me through, or a hammer pounding on my head, or the tissues being ripped and torn apart, the conjuring of these images suggests that the patient is no longer able to tolerate the pain and this is a matter without quantitation of the pain.

This situation is hard to present to the patient who is suffering and who has a bias against others who are labeled as having psychological amplification of their pain problem. This is a lack of information regarding chronic pain and the problem of unrealistic expectations, perhaps because of media presentations of new medical treatments, which always result in a flocking of patients for a new miracle cure. The information taught by the back school advising a patient how to lift, how to put the laundry into the washing machine, how to push the sweeper, how to rake the leaves in the yard, how to stand at the bench and perform tasks for the industrial factory worker, and so forth, is information that requires a significant time commitment that a physician cannot be expected to provide in the office without props and, thus, is not being conveyed. Nonetheless, we have to realize that these patients come to a doctor for help and sometimes are sent to a specialist or even a surgeon for back pain. These patients are not known to that specialist; and, particularly, that specialist may be a surgeon who is completely unfamiliar with the environment and job situation and particularly, the stress with which this patient comes preconditioned, either for success or failure. Such background would perhaps give a valuable perspective to guide their treatment, but this information is primarily available to the primary caretaker for this patient. I thus assert that the primary care physician needs to become more familiar with the totality of low back care as a valued member of the rehabilitation team, not capitulating to the captain of the ship, the spine surgeon, without at least transmitting as best as possible this background information. Unfortunately, some surgeons neglect to make best use of the information and fail to reinforce the primary care practitioner's awareness of the appropriateness and need for his involvement.

We would suggest that low back pain in this setting would suggest the need for greater active involvement in physical fitness; and, particularly, exercises such as swimming are excellent for back problems and should be recommended. Swimming allows the reduction of stresses across the spine because of the buoyancy of the water. Flexibility is encouraged in the water because of the ease of movement, and the jarring that is commonly present in jogging is avoided. Jogging is the most common activity for physical conditioning but may aggravate, through heel strike, problems in the spine by the impact and vibration as opposed to walking in which at least one foot is on the ground at all times.

We have followed through the progression that has been commonly seen in orthopedic surgery, and medicine in general, as the field of sports medicine. The purpose of this book is partly to translate the concepts that have been so readily adapted into the care of the knee, shoulder, hip, elbow, and ankle into the care of the neck and lower back, which seems to be slower in coming around to concepts of fitness and active participation in rehabilitation. This new area of sports medicine involves the care of patients who have recreational injuries, and for which they are being treated so that they will remain capable of competing. This departs from previous levels of satisfaction or attention in medical care. That is, if a patient had a broken limb or an injured joint, and if they could walk and work, that is all that would be expected. However, with the enormous sums being paid to professional athletes, and the even greater number of recreational athletes committed to various sports, a higher standard of care has emerged. Patients are now expected to be able to return to the playing field and to perform competitively or even on an elite basis following major disruption of joints and bones. Although we may differentiate the level of competitiveness, this extends to recreation that is no longer an option or alternate leisure activity, but becomes part of a general fitness and longevity program that patients pursue as a matter of good health and fitness. We are no longer concentrating on the disease model, but we are talking about the best possible bodily physiologic function being conditioned and trained, as in competitive athletics, for a more enjoyable career and for participation in leisure, which should increase our longevity, our capability and clarity of mind, for example, from a healthy body, on the job as well. The Greek philosophers would presumably be proud of our "discovery" of this matter that they felt so strongly about so long ago.

As we move away from the disease model and just fixing things that are broken into preventative medicine, reconditioning, and returning to the high level of physiologic function, we need to recognize a greater involvement on the part of the patient in many areas. Back pain is a situation that involves active involvement on the part of the patient. Recovery from many back problems involves exercise, restoration of muscle tone, good overall health, and general fitness through exercise, good posture, and lifting methods. Physicians can prescribe exercise programs, but compliance involves active participation on the part of the patient. It is unfortunate that the sincere attempt on the part of some patients to do exactly what the doctor says, but passively, may prevent them from aggressively rehabilitating their back. In fact, some patients are afraid to move or do almost anything until they check with their doctor. This is laudable in terms of the historical model of disease and being cared for by the doctor, but when we are talking about conditions of fitness or good health, it is common as a sports medicine doctor to be giving advice to the patient rather than specific prohibitions or restrictions. That is, the patient tries to do what he can, and when it hurts, he continues to the limit of his tolerance. He will not peremptorily ask the doctor whether he can perform a certain function, but will test the limits in matters of endurance and even customarily to the point of severe pain. This is what distinguishes the athlete.

One common problem is that many patients find the notion of exercise incredulous. That is, a manual laborer who works hard and has very strong muscles with the endurance to work through an eight-hour or longer day thinks the doctor who presumably does not swing a hammer, carry boxes, or lift weights does not have any perception of what real manual work is, and, hence, is out in left field when exercises are recommended. Similarly, the housewife who comes in with back pain and spends her day picking up laundry, changing diapers, changing beds, sweeping, carrying kids, and many other activities, finds the doctor who prescribes exercises to someone exerting that much activity and manual function to be less than credible, particularly in terms of understanding how much they are doing. Exercise, indeed, is a medicine that doesn't seem to taste bad enough to be appropriate for my <u>severe</u> pain; but, as presented in the last chapter, surgery is for nerve compression which is correlated with a specific examination as well as imaging studies like an MRI and, specifically, not with the perceived severity of the problem or even of the pain. Before exercise is instituted, attention needs to be directed to posture, as well as lifting techniques and body mechanics for the injured worker. The young mother may be more receptive to considering these matters as her life has changed dramatically, whereas the carpenter or other manual laborer may feel insulted at the suggestion that he has been lifting or working improperly all his previous career.

If we consider the extension exercises that have been popularized as part of an extensive evaluation and treatment program by Robin MacKenzie, a manipulative physical therapist from New Zealand, we become aware that certain positions of the spine are not achieved in normal daily function. If we stand up straight, that is the neutral position. If we bend over and touch our toes, we are in a flexed position(Figure 6). If we sit in a chair, our knees are bent, but we have returned to the flexed position. If we consider arching our back into extension (Figure 7), we are visualizing a position that has no specific function and is not commonly done during the course of a day. As a consequence, we may have some insight as to why the facet joints are not healthy during a portion of their range of

motion, and in that unhealthy portion, may be irregular on the joint surfaces and catch or elicit marked pain (facet syndrome). Further, the lack of
motion through normal activity from our daily routines, if diminished, will
fail to fully nourish the discs whose nutrition is dependent upon water and
its associated nutritional dissolved materials in the body being drawn in
and extruded out by motions of the spine. So, even for the otherwise physically fit, exercise and posture modifications may be helpful and beneficial.

Often, the spine surgeon will see patients who are unable to participate
in a cardiac rehabilitation program because of concomitant back problems
which prevent them from walking or exercising, for example, on a tread-
mill. This represents a deviation from the standard of care for their heart;
and for best treatment, they may need to undergo other therapeutic inter-
ventions from a back standpoint to participate customarily in the cardiac
program. The situation has extended to the fact that some patients have had
surgery to be better able to walk and exercise for a pain that they would
have otherwise tolerated, but which was part of their cardiac rehabilitation
program. The practical question we might then consider is: a disability or
occupational injury to the spine, where recovery from that injury requires
active participation and extensive rehabilitation on the part of the patient,
is the worker on duty or working at his craft during the participation time
when straining at the weights of the exercise machines to recondition a
recently operated spine? Is the professional athlete on duty when rehabilitating their recently operated knee? Is the patient in cardiac rehabilitation,
disabled by injury to the heart, back at work in the same sense when doing
walking and cardiac rehabilitation exercises? By analogy then, is the factory worker who has sustained an injury to the back by slipping on a wet or
greasy floor actually on duty or starting a return-to-work when they participate in a painful and vigorous work-hardening program prescribed by
the doctor?

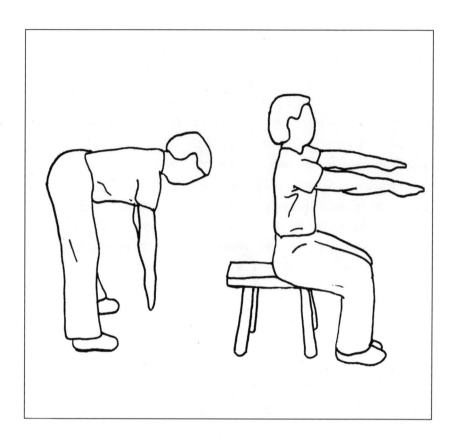

Figure 6

Bending over to touch the toes is the same to the spine position as being seated in a chair.

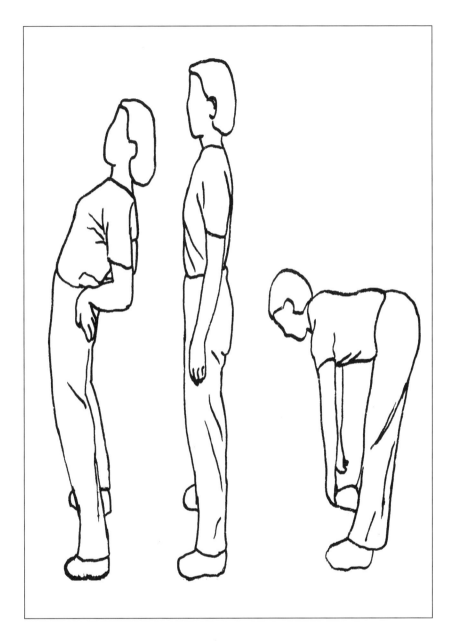

Figure 7

Full range of motion of the lumbar spine includes forward flexion and backward bending; arching extends the spine, a position that is not customarily achieved during normal activities.

Perhaps many readers would suggest, as some of my patients have, that what happens when the insurance carrier decides to terminate benefits, seek a minimum cost settlement, and refuses to provide funds or authorization for physical therapy (which relieves pain, at least to some extent) is that the employees are actually working for their employer as well as themselves when they are trying to get back to work by rehabilitating. Further, the insurance carrier's refusal to reimburse these costs while therapy still holds the prospect of restoring the employee's function and employability, is difficult to understand since it is in the interest of the employer in many cases. It is in those cases, usually the contention of the insurance carrier based upon past experience in general and not with respect to this specific patient, that these treatments, such as physical therapy, are no longer therapeutic in the sense that they lead to recovery, but are maintenance in the sense that they only relieve pain. This may often be the case after extended treatments, either with physical therapists who continue to see the patient and actually provide diminishing attention, only providing hot packs or other modalities, or some chiropractors who seem to fail to discharge the patient who is not progressing. Part of the medical system is to relieve pain; and it is hard to understand how an effective treatment, even if it did not lead to 100 percent recovery and return to work, full recovery is not always feasible, how that can be considered a criterion for the insurance carrier's obligations under the law. On the other hand, pain and suffering of the disabled are disallowed since this is not a tort situation. So, rehabilitation is covered but palliation may not be.

Nonetheless, the patient may actually wait years without treatment, at which point results are expected to diminish as legal maneuvering tests the patient's resolve to hold out for a maximum settlement. For example, one of my patients was referred by me to a physician affiliated with a particular rehabilitation program that I felt held the possibility that the patient could return to light duty with subsequent return to productivity, self-esteem, and eventually be off the compensation roles. That referral was denied by the insurance carrier, who slightly more than one year later sent the patient a registered letter demanding that he report to a physician of his choice for an examination. The physician to whom they were demanding he appear under threat of termination of benefits and legal repercussions, was the same physician to whom I had referred them but who had been refused. That physician subsequently evaluated the patient and then that physician recommended the treatment protocol which I had earlier sought. That recommendation obtained as a result of the insurance carrier's extreme coercion, was denied by the adjuster selecting that physician. This treatment was thought by the rehabilitation physician, who was first my choice and then the insurance carrier's choice, to help the patient and now whose potential for returning to work was dependent upon these recommendations that were denied. Perhaps it is the belief by this employer that this patient was abusing the system; but this is not an objective, unbiased viewpoint, because the employer does have a clearly identifiable interest which should include the ability of the patient to do some work, and an obligation to bring rehabilitation resources to the patient for maximal medical improvement. Further, the employee would be continuing to cooperate with physical therapy that has been ordered under the prescription of the patient's physician. The other contention would be that the insurance carrier might find a loophole to say that this was not truly a job-related injury, but just an arthritic or age-related condition, and some medical examiner has opined that they should not be liable. Unfortunately, that opinion is by a one-time examiner which is not as influential objectively as the treating physician who sees the patient periodically for follow-up and treatment, and some of these examiners are so predictable in their opinions that their objectivity is no longer credible.

As we consider problems in the low back, we need to keep in perspective the need for physical fitness, as well as the need to treat empiricall. We need to deal with problems even when we are not specifically aware of a pathoanatomic lesion (we can't point to the exact cause), and to recognize that the disability is the actual problem for which we may require other health professionals in a coordinated fashion, such as a functional restoration treatment plan that in its complete form can provide maximum treatment and return the patient to satisfactory function. Certainly when some patients are sent to physical therapy they feel that their problem is not appreciated for its severity and that they could have done those exercises on their own anyway. This attitude may be unrealistic; they may not be able to achieve an effective physical therapy and reconditioning program without supervision, and this is really an anticipation that the physician's prescription cannot work because the medicine simply doesn't taste bad enough. Although some patients may be able to rehabilitate themselves effectively from an exercise instruction sheet or their general awareness, having been in a health club, aerobic program, or some other fitness program, an advantage of supervised physical therapy is that it can also give the physician feedback about the patient's cooperation, attitudes, or even depression, all of which affect the outcome. This information allows the physician then to direct subsequent physical therapy specifically and insure that the patient has instruction in posture, lifting techniques, or even back school, as well as any other specific needs of that particular patient that can be identified. Nonetheless, physical fitness can be extremely effective, particularly when it is recognized by patients as the beginning of a process that they will continue indefinitely, recognizing that exercise is its own reward and they are becoming more actively involved in their recovery and subsequently in their fitness or good health. The psychological benefits that result from fitness were highly publicized and evident in the jogging rage of a few years ago. Unfortunately, jogging seems to jar the spine whereas swimming would be much more effective in promoting flexibility and muscular conditioning in addition to buoyancy in the water relieving the stress of gravity from the spine.

"Exercise is its own reward" should be our motto. Perhaps we should question whether exercise in many senses is a treatment or patient responsibility. Clearly this is a matter of our concept of being treated (passive) or the physician diagnosing the problem requiring (active) participation. This includes some means such as physical therapy which require a prescription that the physician is uniquely empowered by law to authorize. This authorization may be a matter of restricting dangerous drugs to supervised medical conditions, or as in the case of back pain, may more commonly represent the need for the physician really to assert in a legal sense that the patient needs this treatment and hence payment is part of the authorized compensable injury. As such, the physician is no longer the gatekeeper of the dangers of medication for the untrained (such as narcotics and other dangerous medication), but the arbiter from an economic standpoint of the medical need for treatments. This is not a need in the sense that a patient who has appendicitis will die without the needed surgery: this is a need in terms of that patient's comfort, lifestyle, productivity, and other essential human factors, but not of survival. Certainly in some cases a depressed, disabled female worker might benefit more from a visit to the hairdresser and a permanent than physical therapy, but I have not as yet written that prescription. It should be self-evident that matters of comfort, lifestyle, productivity, and so forth are certainly necessary, but the extent to which they should be provided becomes extraordinarily subjective on the part of the individual practitioner called upon to make these decisions. Beyond subjectivity and the fact that this is not medical care in a traditional sense in which the doctor was trained, the physician is put in the middle and can never please both parties, and is likely to become the target of frustration for both.

People feel better, have less pain, and are less susceptible to injury when they are in good condition. Endorphins are created when we are exercising and not only are our minds cleared by a good sweat from aerobic exercise, but our capacity to do other activities is increased by the exertion. This is true for patients with back pain and, in fact, many of the problems with pain may simply be matters of deconditioning or lack of normal exercise. It is unfortunate that some of the deconditioning may be a result of historically accepted medical treatment. Soldiers on the battlefield certainly have the ability to survive and to fight without noticing some wounds or pain which are only a small part of their awareness until they reach the hospital, because their attention is so concentrated on survival on the battlefield that their mind doesn't have space to give attention to these other problems. Similarly, the marathon runner is concentrating on victory and some have even crossed the finish line on broken bones, which hurt only after concluding the race.

Expectations of modern medicine are a difficult problem to deal with. From the standpoint of sports medicine, many patients with a significant disruption of a knee ligament may be candidates for surgical repair of that ligament. Unfortunately, the rehabilitation that is mandatory for a good result may be beyond the realistic expectations for many patients. While we are impressed to see an elite athlete return to high-level function following a surgical intervention, we are not aware, perhaps, of the extent of the commitment and pain endured in the rehabilitation for a good result to occur.

Certainly we have recognized in the treatment of certain fractures that it is no longer acceptable to place these in a cast indefinitely until the bone heals and then look upon the X ray of a healed bone as a success. If, in fact, the joint is so scarred from the fracture, the hemorrhage, and the inflammation, and worse, from the immobilization, inactivity, and loss of use from being in the cast, then it may be basically useless for athletic function or even for many customary activities. It is no longer acceptable to say, "It was a bad fracture." We are now able to use internal fixation, plates, rods, screws, and wires to stabilize the bones so that activities such as joint motion can occur promptly, before this irreparable disease which is called by the Swiss Society for Internal Fixation, "cast disease," occurs. When I visited China, I was introduced to the Zen treatment of fractures: the polar opposites of mobilization and immobilization were brought together (by bamboo splints) to stabilize the bone and mobilize the joints and brought into the dynamic harmony of the path. Unfortunately, it is still a recommendation of some physicians that patients are at bed rest as an important treatment in backache. Hospitalized in-patient care is a form of enforced bed rest under the impression that effectiveness requires strict bedrest and that traction, otherwise available at home through visiting nurse organizations, and traction equipment is really just an enforcement of bed rest. Further, it is carte blanche ordered for each recurrent episode or worsened experience of pain. Studies have shown that prolonged bed rest is not effective and, particularly, it is not effective in longer stretches than two days. As such, the treatment interferes with recovery, but this is the objective scientific basis offered in the literature, which is at variance with the emotional attachment that physicians have to treatments that give excellent results for that disease during spontaneous resolution, as ninety percent are recovered without treatment within three months.

Physicians are often frustrated with the lack of benefit in disabled patients of effective treatments when rendered in noncompensation patients, with or without surgery. A particular patient may seek to have her back pain and disability relieved only to find that her boss does not understand and is just as mean and demanding as ever, and that insurance company that didn't want to pay for her necessary medical care after all of her loyal years with the company. This can be very threatening and reveal the company's lack of appreciation of this contributing employee. I recall a patient who was admitted to a detoxification program having already had complete elimination of the back pain through a specialized surgical procedure. At that time, prior to MRI, epidural venograms were used to detect disc ruptures when myelogram with CT scan was indeterminate. He had that procedure followed by a microdiscectomy and complete relief of the leg pain for which he had been taking medication and other treatments. This pilot of a commercial airliner was troubled ethically and morally by the recognition that the prescription drugs (Percocet) that he had been obtaining were actually an addiction and he was unable to avoid them even though the back pain was totally eliminated. He was literally flying high prior to signing in to a detoxification program at risk of his profession. The difficulty on the part of the practitioner is how to deal with the patient who accuses the physician of not understanding or caring by refusing to provide addictive narcotics for the severe pain, even after multiple explanations of the fact that it is a chronic problem. For a longstanding chronic problem, addictive narcotics are contraindicated, leading to enormous problems. Not only is the addiction an additional problem, not part of the first problem, but it is a problem for which the physician is at least partly culpable, and in particular, beyond the drug addiction, leads to a physician dependence type of addiction and perpetuation of the illness or passivity.

Many patients will benefit from any treatment offered until the point comes when it is suggested that return to work should be shortly possible. At that point, no treatment can be effective as we recall some of the job stresses or problems which had previously occurred. We often see the patient act as if he were going to leave the back at the therapist's establishment and pick it up in three weeks when it was fixed. In many cases the lack of benefit is a consequence of lack of active involvement on the patient's part; and although I hope not to be misunderstood, specifically, I am not accusing patients who fail to benefit as being at fault for their lack of benefit. However, every patient who becomes more actively involved in one's care will be better off because of the commitment and participation in the prescribed treatment. It is the patient's back problem and the patient is the one who will benefit. That is, following the prescription is still a tenet of medical philosophy and care, but actively following it rather than passively is essential where the low back is involved.

Hence, physicians look selectively for disc problems because our treatment is so good for that problem and we are a little reluctant to settle on calling the problem a facet syndrome when (a) we can't prove it, and (b) we can't definitively and decisively treat it. Unfortunately, asymptomatic patients will have abnormalities of the disc on discograms, myelograms, CT scans, and MRI. These may appear to be operable lesions and, in fact, may have unnecessary surgery recommended. As a consequence, the patient then has a scar on top of the previous problem, is without relief, and the actual problem may have been missed. This patient may even be recommended another operation to fix the problem, presuming again that it must be a disc problem. Many times the interpretation of the MRI, or myelogram, or CT scan will have the definitive qualifier, "clinical correlation needed." That is to say, if the patient has a disc, the meaning of the anatomic situation seen on the imaging study has to be confirmed by examination of pain location, factors that ameliorate or exacerbate, and confirming neurologic signs. If, for example, the problem is a facet problem, and an asymptomatic disc is present in MRI, because there is pain and some irritation of the nerve from the facet joint causing pain to go into the leg, the likelihood of an unnecessary disc operation is substantial. It is certainly self-evident that an appendectomy will not help gall bladder disease, even though we are providing an effective and well-established treatment for abdominal pain.

Following this analogy further, patients not only need to have an active role in rehabilitation and understand the need to overcome the passive trusting role that has been encouraged for centuries, but again in parallel with sports medicine, they need to become participatory in their treatment. That is, if a patient has an anterior cruciate tear and is a competitive athlete, surgery might be indicated. If they are not a high-level competitive person, then treatment with muscle rehabilitation without surgery may be an appropriate consideration for them. It clearly is a sports medicine doctor's obligation to present to the patient fairly and reasonably the options based upon current medical literature. Though the literature is being written every day and is significantly changing, but assuming the physician is up to date, information should be available for the patient to make an informed choice. The choice then has to be made with patients who have back problems who, for example, have pain and may be unable to function at their prior level, but would be better off to return to work than to have an operation for poor surgical indications. That is, a small disc without clearly pinching a nerve and the subsequent symptoms of a pinched nerve, even with a bulging or injured disc on MRI, may provide the patient with some relief. But, that patient must be forewarned that they may have some relief but not be able to return to high-level manual activities, such as heavy lifting, solely as a result of that surgery. If they are to return to that heavy-duty job, they might have insignificant improvement by the operation but require major change through rehabilitation and exercise.

The best course may often be to defer the surgery if it is not going to change one's status and allow the patient to return to limited work as one would otherwise, unless the patient is willing to go through the exercise program that may be more beneficial. The easiest avenue is for the patient to accept limitations that one may have; if still with those limitations, surgery is desired, then it is an informed decision and thus becomes appropriate with optimization of one's other overall function by the postoperative rehabilitation. Unfortunately, many physicians who are eager to do the surgery with an unjustified pride in their own work (or failure to appreciate the number of other surgeons who also do good work) or anticipation of an unusually good result on a fortuitous basis, urge the patient to have a procedure that may make them better but does not relieve the entire problem. The appropriate sequence would be for that patient to have reasonable recommendations based upon the exam and imaging studies and the specific demands of one's job. As the demand of a particular athlete's sport, we should reasonably be able to predict the likelihood of a patient returning to heavy lifting after a disc injury or other spinal problem and should so inform the patient, so that he can actively not only make a decision, but be involved in a rehabilitation program that should be part of the insurance carrier's approval prior to embarking upon the surgical procedure. The patient who deteriorates after surgery from a fitness standpoint because the insurance carrier is disputing whether the injury is actually their liability and whether it might have been a nonwork-related problem or whether they can just return to work without the expense of rehabilitation resources should be anticipated prior to embarking upon surgery, with the consent of the patient to acquire his active participation as well as specific information from the surgeon and the understanding of the insurance carrier of the plan proposed. Having presented the need for active participation in a program, we would like to turn our attention to the aspects of an appropriate comprehensive program that can meet the needs of industrial injuries or compensation patients.

Chapter 5

PROGRAM

Unfortunately, in the real practice of spine care, rehabilitation techniques are often confused with conservative care, with the use of passive or invasive physical modalities remaining the rule well after a period of soft tissue healing. Often, passive modalities are incorporated into efforts at functional restoration by well-meaning clinicians unclear as to the guidelines prohibiting such treatments as contraindicated.

—Robert J. Gatchel, et al, *Spine*, 1992

Many people are not content with their weight, and thus it is a common practice to be on a diet. Technically, we could say that everyone is on a diet, as the description of what is eaten is your diet. If you eat nothing, you are on a starvation diet! As we consider the problem of being overweight and how common this problem actually is, we recognize that there are an enormous number of people who are on a weight-reduction diet. As we consider diets of many kinds, we come away with a perspective, after we have reviewed the exaggerated claims of many programs and gimmicks, and by common sense, come to the need for caloric restriction and exercise as the basis for not only good health but an appropriate diet. Good fitness requires good aerobic exercise which, to some extent, causes appetite suppression by generating ketones in our system. This prevents us from overeating and helps control caloric intake without undue hunger while burning some of the calories that we have already eaten.

Returning to the problems of the back, there are no lack of promises or gimmicks for the relief of back pain. The previous chapter was intended to emphasize a balanced position in analogy to a diet coupled with exercise and active involvement of the patient. Beyond the lack of patient teaching about back pain on the part of physicians, what actually are the physicians taught? I am impressed with the empiric nature of the informal and limited instruction that I received in treating low back pain while I was in medical school, internship, and residency training. Namely, that low back pain was treated with bed rest and certain medications, perhaps physical therapy and/or traction. Traction has not been shown to be beneficial on an objective basis and in the past it was at least unofficially considered as a justification to bring a patient into the hospital. This could conveniently increase the expense of spinal injury to arbitrary limits that might be set by no-fault laws and thus make it a litigatable no-fault claim. It also accommodated the convenience of the physician who could then evaluate the patient while making rounds on other patients in the hospital on a daily basis and with all of the test results and other information conveniently summarized in the hospital chart. Many of us are familiar with patients who are sent to some physicians by their attorney with a recommendation that they need to be hospitalized or placed in traction. Unfortunately, this left the patient in a passive dependent role. Namely, nothing is being done by the patient except to wait for the physician to cure them or to heal them. Not only is this a passive role for the patient, but the physician is really waiting for the passage of time, which we would interpret as resolution of swelling from an injury or inflammation from a flare of a preexisting problem by providing a therapy that is now available at home. Further, body muscle mass can deteriorate up to three percent per day at bed rest; and, hence, an enormous deficit can occur by the end of two weeks, which certainly would aggravate any spine problem or, in fact, may cause de novo pain in many patients. Nonetheless, this passive treatment still is standard for many physicians. The information to follow in this chapter exceeds medical instruction that I had received and may exceed the knowledge of many practitioners.

Many studies have been presented in the literature, as part of evidence-based medicine, which considers the various treatments, all of which are available for patients with back pain. In fact, these studies have shown that most of the medical treatments are ineffective. Even the proponents of manipulation have failed to show after a course of six weeks of treatment any continued further benefit for those being manipulated, as opposed to patients not offered that treatment, or upon whom sham manipulation (not actually performing a manipulation) is performed. On the other hand, chiropractic care statistically returns patients to work sooner than traditional medical care by M.D.s. In early (less than three weeks) treatment there seems to be some advantage to manipulation, but the advantage is lost with increasing time and not of such great magnitude as to be thus far demonstrated by the many prospective randomized controlled (scientific) studies attempting to establish the role and value of manipulation for chronic low back pain or sciatica. Unfortunately, the natural history of this disease is so good that spontaneous recovery can easily be blamed upon a treatment that happened to be offered. Certainly if ninety percent of patients will be completely better in three months without treatment, a treatment that did not make the patient worse, would therefore give a ninety percent excellent result within three months. An uncritical attitude would say that this is an excellent treatment even though it is totally ineffective. Practitioners would demand that this treatment be offered, that it was medically necessary, and that it was the standard of care and certainly must be used and could not be denied the patient because of such outstanding results, misinterpreting the results of spontaneous recovery and natural history.

This is particularly true with the problem of backache. When patients are not content because of their pain, they have heard of the excellent treatments many of their friends or work associates have received. Thus, they seek medical attention rather than exercising for good health with a problem that almost universally recovers but they also are in need of documentation for their disability. We need to be careful and acknowledge by and large that the passage of time with active involvement and gradual resumption of activity is the most effective treatment available, and that cannot be taken for granted. Further, the spine needs to be fit and healthy, which requires not only a brief period of rest after injury, but the resumption of activities and careful progressive use of muscles not only to stretch out the formerly swollen tissues, but to increase appropriate blood flow and normal muscle tone for good health and for resumption of normal function. We are often surprised to appreciate the meticulous prolonged exercise programs that are required to regain the elusive matters of endurance and work or exercise tolerance, which is surprisingly quickly lost and astonishingly slow to be recovered. This is, however, the same as calf muscle bulk lost while in a cast for a fractured ankle or in the thigh after knee surgery.

In this chapter we will discuss the various forms of treatment available. As we suggest in an escalating manner the types of treatment available starting with simpler ones and proceeding through a menu of modalities and treatments, we are presenting in sequence the treatments that would be offered to a progressively worse back pain problem. If we have a few pounds to lose, an increase in exercise such as taking a walk at lunchtime may be sufficient. If we are considering a diet for a large weight reduction program, then we may need a combination of not only severe caloric restriction, medical follow-up and monitoring, but also supervised exercises and perhaps some equipment. As the problem becomes more severe, the solution becomes more complex and a sufficient program needs to be instituted. Unfortunately, if we have a severe problem and an inadequate solution, the conclusion is often drawn, "I can't lose weight." That is patently false and we know that without eating, no person will magically gain weight by breathing air or drinking plain water and that every living organism will lose weight. We also know that the amount of calories taken and the amount of exercise or other consumption of calories will determine how much weight is retained, gained, or lost. There are no mysteries, but we certainly will find it difficult to lose weight without exercise and many programs such as Weight Watchers and others have clearly demonstrated the value of behavioral modification as an integral part of any successful weight control program.

If we are considering a disability, then we have a problem that may require multidisciplinary resources. For success in difficult cases, a complete pain or functional restoration program may be required and will be described in this chapter. Unfortunately, if the therapies described and suggested here are incompletely available, then success for some patients is not as reliably predicted, as it would be for the comprehensive program. It is only for the comprehensive program that we by analogy with either dieting or with low back pain would anticipate effectiveness for the individual who has serious problems. If caloric intake restriction is coupled with medical follow-up and supervision, as well as specific exercise and a complete behavioral or psychological support program, then success is far more reliable than when a sheet is given just listing foods and their caloric values and relying upon the patient to use this sheet consistently, to understand it fully, and to modify behavior without exception in compliance with its recommendations.

It is in the same sense necessary that a comprehensive rehabilitation program be made available for difficult cases or we will be dealing with the ineffectiveness of portions of a treatment program which in and of themselves are effective for simple cases, but does not mean that the patient cannot benefit from treatment, but rather that inadequate facilities have been made available. That is, we will have a therapeutic failure because the appropriate complete program and treatment are not provided to the individual, as it was needed. Clearly this is analogous again to the weight control programs that are often available where we see innumerable gimmicks promoted as the answer to a weight control problem without all of the difficult problems of calorie restriction and exercises as if someone had found a magic answer. It seems self-evident that there is no magic answer, or everyone would be promptly following this new revolutionary method. Such a revolutionary method is not really available, but common sense with caloric restriction and exercise does lead to weight control. Unfortunately, the lack of success without the complete program gives rise to a host of excessive claims and incredible techniques or devices, as burning fat without being hungry and so forth. There certainly is no lack of facilities for patients with low back pain and practitioners, many of whom make extraordinary claims. Of these, I am most irritated by the "complete" programs that lack the resources and expertise to accomplish the task, leaving the patient as a failure due to an inadequate program rather than their actual back pain problem.

Following is an outline of the menu from which as complete a program as necessary could be selected, or alternately as little as is necessary can be provided for other cases that do not require all of these component parts. Certainly the majority of backaches do not receive medical attention, as they are better spontaneously with the passing of time without seeing a doctor. The patient has assumed it will go away and subsequently has gradually resumed all activities, effectively rehabilitating as necessary. When injuries do come to the attention of a physician, health coordinator, exercise physiologist, chiropractor, or others, we can self-treat with aspirin, hot packs or hot showers, and simple exercises in an attempt to reduce some of the inflammation or swelling and pain, and have the difficult residual left for professional treatment. As we introduce a progressively more invasive program, we need to continue to use minimal treatment for cases that will resolve with time and patience, but we cannot cure all problems by going to physical therapy without work hardening, functional restoration, and comprehensive pain management programs for other cases that require those resources to restore the patient who has failed initially effective treatments to return to normal function. We should keep in mind that the principal effect is to reduce inflammation or the swelling, albeit through various means. The next step beyond reducing swelling is surgery.

BED REST

Bed rest has been around since the Egyptians and continues to be an important part of treatment. Bed rest longer than two days has been shown by objective studies to be no more effective than two days and as a consequence we would recommend the limitation of bed rest as much as possible. The rest position or what has been termed the first-aid position for the back really represents an attempt to find a pain-free posture. This may differ in some cases, but usually when in bed, most pain will be relieved. Patients who continue to have problems or spasm will find that elevating the knees such that the hips and knees are flexed will result in further relief of pain. Some patients find that by lying on the floor with their legs up on a chair, giving them 90° at the hip and knee, they are in a completely pain-free position. When a new attack of back pain comes and the patient has been functioning normally for an interval, return to bedrest or the first aid position may be helpful. We would further recommend that prolonging bed rest beyond the point where the patient feels somewhat comfortable in bed or at least there is some reduction in muscle spasm is inappropriate for the back joints, as for any other joints or parts of the musculoskeletal system.

The common situation is where a patient calls and complains that they are much, much worse, and either requests to be seen immediately by the doctor, to have habituating narcotic medication, desire to be admitted or

X-rayed, and basically just "want something done." These patients may have been followed by the physician, whom they are now calling, for several years, but have had no episode or trauma that would signify an acute change, but it is not possible in today's medicolegal climate to exclude the possibility of a disc rupture, progression toward neurologic compromise, or even the eventual need for surgery resulting from a problem that may occur without a clearly identified antecedent cause. Further, they have been brought into the office on an emergency basis on a number of occasions and nothing was observed on examination to warrant that treatment, so it is probably like crying wolf.

As a consequence, it is easy to recommend observation; that is, the patient is restricted in activities by medical prescription, to bed for rest. This is safe for the physician, since the patient is not likely to worsen objectively or the physician feel liable if there is nerve injury from a disc pressing on a nerve that has not been appreciated because the patient was not immediately seen. Having cried "wolf," ten times in the last three months, one of those times can be a problem but being at bed rest at least would not make it worse. The failure to obtain imaging studies or other expensive examination or even hospital admission could be a problem on any one particular occasion, but after multiple complaints without trauma of worsening, it certainly is not appropriate to continue overtreating. Certainly being told by your doctor that you have to go to bed because the pain is so bad certifies to your family members and others who have to assist with daily chores that you are in too much pain to remain responsible for housework or returning to the job. On the other hand, we might consider bed rest in some senses as a test; a tumor will generally feel worse at bed rest and will keep the patient awake or awakened from sleep, so that raises some concerns. Patients who cannot sleep, as contrasted with those who are awakened from sleep, are seldom afflicted with a physical problem in the back but rather have what would be described as anxiety or difficulty coping with either the pain or the limitations in their activities that it represents. Even patients after spinal surgery with severe pain get to sleep, but patients who complain about pain twenty-four hours a day certainly have to be considered to be exaggerating and trying to emphasize how bad the problem is for the physician's appreciation of how much they need help. Patients who are anxious because of their inability to cope with the back and particularly their inability to return to their normal activities will develop insomnia which is a matter of anxiety, even though there may be pain present to which the sleeplessness is attributed. I regard the patient who repeatedly tells me of the inability to sleep to emphasize the severity of pain as a patient who is in distress because of the pain, and this is what we would technically call a pain behavior or illness behavior rather than a true gauge of pain severity.

Having prescribed bed rest as management for the patient who is otherwise demanding narcotics or habituating medication for a problem that has shown itself not to be a short-term one, which will resolve, such as post-surgical pain for which narcotics are appropriate, the treatment of bed rest may be causing a perpetuation of the disability as well as encouraging the development of support systems for the patient at home who is necessarily cared for as if they are unable to get out of bed, or in some cases, in the hospital. In most cases, in retrospect, it is clear that the patient was unable to cope rather than having a solely physical problem. Nonetheless, the experience of pain was real, severe, and demanded attention of some sort, although certainly narcotic addiction is a problem rather than a help, and in fact, addiction to inactivity is a damaging treatment if overused. I can cite examples of many patients who, between monthly visits, have shown up in the emergency room, totally incapacitated and requiring intramuscular injections of narcotics, as they are unable to live or sleep or function at all because of the total attention their disability and pain problem has resulted in. I recall a patient in particular who, on four occasions ,was in the emergency room, and when I saw him in the office I asked about his physical problem, whether or not the insurance company had accepted his proposed settlement offer. In fact, I had correctly assessed the situation and found that his perspective of it and his ability to deal with the pain had become compromised by intransigence on the insurer's part and the loss of the glimmer of hope that he had received from that proposed settlement.

Bed rest is an effective treatment and a valuable part of our armamentarium, whether for backache or for the common cold. We know after the common cold that we have to get up and get our strength back after the inactivity, and thus we must be careful to avoid overprescribing bed rest.

Clearly, as the main benefit is to reduce muscle spasm and allow edema to resolve, there is no magical or mystical component to being at rest in bed. Scientifically, the disc pressure has been measured and is significantly less at bed rest and thus we would expect that an acute disc herniation, which presses on a nerve and causes sciatica, would have less pressure on the nerve and thus less pain into the leg while at bed rest. The problem is that most back injuries are not acute disc ruptures; in fact, 98 percent do not involve symptoms suggesting sciatica. Further, any exacerbation of the preexisting problem should not automatically be advised to seek relief with bed rest as this may become an addictive, self-defeating, and pain-perpetuating cycle.

MODALITIES

Medical recommendations following any injury generally recommend adding ice to the affected area, or if it is a chronic problem, using heat to soothe swollen muscles or inflamed areas. Physical therapy has included many new ways to apply heat, some of which are effective and gratifying to the patient troubled by problems with the back. The application of heat by moist hot packs is time honored, and because of better contact with the skin, moist heat will not only penetrate deeper, but also have less risk of burning the surface of the skin by transferring heat. In addition, deeper heating, or diathermy can be accomplished with ultrasound or with electromagnetic energy, although the latter is less commonly used today. Electrical stimulation is commonly used where muscles are stimulated by an electric current, either through electrodes or as part of the ultrasound transducer, in which muscles are stimulated to contract, increasing blood flow, reducing spasm, along with heating by the ultrasound mechanical signal.

Today, counterirritants are available as a variety of lotions and other rub-on ointments, as well as a battery pack for transcutaneous electrical stimulation (TENS) which, for considerable expense, produces a buzz, that is less disagreeable than pain. In addition, tight muscles may be massaged and the knots worked out of them. A technique of myofascial release has been developed out of recognition that the muscles and fascia are three-dimensional and after an injury may be in a contracted or tight state. Many of the complaints of patients are exactly that they feel tight, and of course, this can be related to their posture by viewing the patient from a slight distance undressed. Clearly, any alteration of normal posture is going to cause a cumulative discomfort through a day's activities and becomes a significant problem, even though most medical education has not regarded the importance of fatigue and functional posture. While therapists perform these therapies, osteopaths have become familiar with this problem and experts in the matter for quite a few years as well as chiropractors who are not overly quick to manipulate but deal with necessary stretching and soft tissue mobilization prior to extending the range of motion of joints or the spine or essentially performing a manipulation. Massage may temporarily exacerbate the pain but usually feels better after a course of treatment. The Greeks thought rheuma, or cold, was the problem, so they essentially did the same thing, as back pain was part of rheumatism. Whether our reasons are better we should never fight results, and certainly heat and counterstimulants help. Our task is to consider the question of whether or not the patient is equally capable of self-treating and applying these remedies without supervision.

Modalities are increasingly used in health spas, by chiropractors, and by other health advocates for relieving tight muscles and the pain of conditioning or exercise. From a theoretical standpoint, when a patient has an injury of an extremity or the spine, the counterirritants have some soothing benefit, but also the use of cold may vasoconstrict to prevent swelling from increasing, or at a later time such as three or four days after injury, heat may alternately be used and is often useful in facilitating the exudation and removal of products of swelling and inflammation through the increased blood flow that occurs from the heat.

Obviously the best way to heat muscles is by exercising them. As a consequence we need to think in terms of the eventual recovery and resumption of function rather than a dependence upon physical therapy. I object to the concept that the physician or physiatrist should order physical therapy at a very specified level for a certain period; for example, three weeks of three times per week of deep heat and ultrasound or 1.5 milliwatts per square centimeter for twenty minutes. The problem is that different patients have different depths of penetration to the muscles, and the issue is heating the muscles to the point that they will be softened so the fascia and ligamentous structures will stretch; and if not, the desired result will not be achieved. I would far prefer that the patient advance to heating the muscles through active involvement in an exercise program as soon as possible rather than waiting to see me at the arbitrary interval having concluded a specified treatment, then be ready for subsequent advancement with further specific restrictive directions. Rather, they should be able to advance as appropriate under the close follow-up of the therapist, either with the modalities or with the actual movement forward into stretching and strengthening exercise. No disease in the body really follows a step or staircase decrease, but heals on a gradual basis, so that as we treat a strep throat, the medication fights the infection with streptococcus and relieves the symptoms within a couple of days. We uniformly emphasize to the patient that they need to complete the full course of treatment for a week or ten days for the specific purpose of totally eradicating the infection rather than having it recur because of inadequate treatment. When the treatment is exercise and normal activity, this is not a necessity that we should specify a fixed interval for the treatment, as it is presumed that work or normal activities will continue to advance fitness, or a home exercise program to follow the supervised physical therapy will maintain the level of fitness achieved.

Unfortunately, physical therapy seems to fall into the mold of other prescribed drugs, that is, needing a specific dose with a prescription like pills, which then reverts back to the passive concept to which I have tried to show the need for active involvement in Chapter III. Further, this limits the physical therapist's independent assessment and expression of skill and capabilities to evaluate and treat on an independent basis the patient who is being seen every day as opposed to the physician seeing the patient on a less frequent basis. In many cases the modalities of hot packs and other physical therapy treatments may be more a matter of hands-on reassurance than actually providing care that is not otherwise available by the patient at home running a towel under hot water and then putting it on the injured area. In addition to reassurance, the combination of exercise instruction and supervision as well as evaluation of response requires supervision.

Modalities can be an effective and important part of the initial management, but have to be limited and converted to active patient involvement or else they can be abused.

MANIPULATION

Certainly manipulation has been historically one of the oldest treatments for back pain and other problems. Having considered the need to resume activities as soon as possible and not lose muscle strength by inactivity, the rationale of any approach that would allow rapid mobilization should be self-evident. Chiropractors and osteopaths have made manipulation a fundamental part of their treatment in varying degrees, and physical therapists in recent years have embarked on more forms of manipulation in their practice, although in many cases it may be stretching exercises and soft tissue mobilization techniques on an active basis by the patient rather than the manual therapist performing manipulation on the patient passively. It is interesting to see, at least from my experience, that many chiropractors have increasingly used the modalities, commonly a part of physical therapy and including mobilization as preceding manipulation, and as a consequence, at least viewed internationally, the professions seem to be merging together for the better treatment of the patient, although they are strictly distinguished in the United States by the fact that physical therapists require a prescription by a physician whereas the chiropractor is an independent practitioner.

Unfortunately, the beneficial effects of manipulation, although they are sudden and gratifying, have not been shown scientifically to contribute reliably or cause further improvement after about six weeks has passed. That is, an enormous number of studies have not shown a difference in patients given manipulation or sham manipulation or no treatment after about six weeks' time; so the treatment should be restricted to either the acute injury within the first few weeks or there is a basis to then consider it a palliative matter, not actually a treatment but a maintenance procedure for pain moderation, and unfortunately, limited by the fact that it is passively done to the patient. Common practice includes many patients who are manipulated chronically, almost as an addiction. Manipulation when it is not for an acute problem does not result in any underlying change or alteration of symp-

toms or disability. As such, it is best part of the initial treatment that is helpful for cases that are understood to be resolving spontaneously and for
which a safe and effective treatment to facilitate recovery and enhance rehabilitation is certainly a helpful adjunct to treatment.

Manipulation is clearly useful for a frozen shoulder and many musculoskeletal physicians will prescribe exercise and perhaps have the patient
receive a general anesthetic and manipulate the shoulder. This process
involves risk of fracturing the bone, but tears scar tissue that is restricting
motion and resulting in pain. The results of increased motion are gratifying,
but the complete resolution of pain requires a subsequent rehabilitation
program. The same should be reasonable for spine problems. Namely,
manipulation should be an effort to initiate an active self-treatment program of exercise and resumption of activity. This is often the case when
manipulation is actively given. On the other hand, chronic manipulation
represents a failure of the patient to resume their normal activities and also
represents a failure of understanding of what the manipulation should provide for the patient. As a physician, my bias is presumably contrary to
manipulation. But having stated that, as well as my previous acceptance of
the usefulness of manipulation within treatment, I would point out that
there is as yet no scientific substantiation of the concept that the disc is actually being manipulated by applied forces; although, there are ongoing studies that suggest the several times body weight would be required for an
acute and forceful thrust to accomodate manipulation. An understanding
of the mechanism of pain relief or of patient improvement from manipulation is suggested from the mechanisms involving the gate control theory of
pain, a distraction mechanism such as the TENS unit, and not from actually putting the bulging disc back in its place. Certainly manipulation of facet
joints causes cavitation and the creation of air bubbles in the joint from sudden expansion. Air bubbles in the facet joints should cushion their motions
and thus restore spinal mobility in a patient who had been restricted by a
facet joint that was locked or inflamed and causing muscle spasm adjacent
to that joint. Certainly MRIs have been shown, before and after manipulation, to have essentially the same anatomic features even with a much-
improved patient from a symptomatic standpoint. A lack of objective scientific basis does not negate the benefits, but it should make us cautious in

subscribing substantial benefit to manipulation, which may otherwise be part of the passing of time and spontaneous improvement from backaches, which do have a good prognosis.

EXERCISES

Exercises are a common part of rehabilitation or medical treatment of back pain, as well as many other musculoskeletal problems. There seems to be some mystery associated with exercises, as if certain ones are inherently dangerous and others are vastly more helpful. Unfortunately, this is part of the gimmickry and mystique of low back programs, the miracle exercises discovered by Dr. What's-his-name. Many patients are particularly concerned about initiating any new activity or starting exercises before they discuss it with their doctor. This artifact of the passive system of being cared for by the all-knowing doctor seems to be yielding to an overall increase in level of information on the public's part, particularly as aerobic exercises are on television incessantly and many people are involved in programs which discuss to some extent the motivation for particular exercises and the concerns and pitfalls in doing such exercises. To be sure that the exercises are performed correctly, effectively, and that the patient is actively involved in putting forth considerable effort, physical therapists can both instruct, assist, and also monitor performance and report back to the physician. Physical therapists seem somewhat reluctant to start new exercises, as they may feel medicolegally liable or being criticized as acting independently if they initiate exercises, or in other cases, for perhaps causing injury. Even though therapists must act on the prescription of a physician, they sometimes demand detailed medical information before they will initiate therapy, in a sense confirming or consenting to the instructions provided or really superseding those instructions, as if acting independently but with the justification of protecting themselves. If we can make the appropriate transition from a passive to an active perspective, everyone with a backache, along with anyone interested in being fit, feeling healthy, and better enjoying their lives, will undertake exercises not only to recover from back problems but be better prepared to handle situations that might otherwise cause further pain.

If we watch an infant awaken, we see the child stretches as we also see our pets often do after a nap. To some extent we all stretch some upon arising after a night's sleep, but many people fail to retain the perspective that an injured spine, no matter how hard a person works or how excellent their state of conditioning, after disability or inability for many weeks or even months, needs to have some stretching as initial exercise. As we look at exercises, I think we should categorize them into mobilizing or stretching exercises, to be followed by strengthening exercises and subsequently reconditioning exercises. This is a clear analogy with the teachings several years ago of Dr. Jack Nickolas, one of the fathers of sports medicine, who suggested that a knee after major surgery should have three months' concentration on range of motion followed by three months of muscular strengthening followed by three months of coordination exercises, the return of proproceptive function, joint position sense function. The spine and associated muscles should first be stretched out to a good range of motion, followed by strengthening and then by endurance or work-tolerance exercises associated with the coordinated activities that are job simulation or realistic for tasks of employment or occupation to be anticipated. (The same order but not the full three-month interval necessarily.)

Considering the stretching exercises, let us review some basic information. I suggest that it is almost intuitive that the spine does not act independently, as most people seem to view it in performing tasks of lifting. As Atlas needed a place to stand to move the earth, so the pelvis needs to be stabilized for the back to have any function in lifting. It has been noted recently in the technical literature that weight lifters, when compared to nonlifters, had stronger and earlier contraction of leg muscles in performing a lift. This is evidently a result of their training, a uniform response, and it has been this physician's experience that patients who have their quadriceps and hamstrings stretched have considerable improvement in their back problems. Strengthening the quadriceps and hamstrings and hip muscles is an essential part of any complete program.

Simplifying exercises conceptually into stretching and relaxation, strengthening, and simulation of real work and reconditioning, we have muscle groups that would be the pelvic girdle, the abdominal muscles, and the erector spinae. Basically there are front muscles, which are flexors of the spine, and those are in the abdomen as well as around the hip. There are muscles that extend the spine during lifting and other activities and these are the erector spinae in the back. Next there are stabilizers of the pelvic girdle or the pelvis upon which the spine rests. These muscles would be the primary foundation, muscles that flex the hip (the iliopsoas), the rectus which is part of the quadriceps mechanism that also extends the knee and the hamstrings that flex the knee but also extend the hip, and the gluteal muscles. It has been estimated that the strength in the muscles that stabilize the pelvic girdle is at least five times greater than the muscles of the back; hence, when the back is inappropriately positioned, serious damage can clearly be seen just by calculating the forces in the muscles for routine lifts in inappropriate positions or with poor technique.

Historically, the common exercises taught for back pain are the flexion exercises (Figure 8) that are intended to increase the tone of the abdominal wall in the anticipation that there will be a greater support for the low back and the spinal column and hence there will be reduced stress on the discs and structures of the low back. The postures described by Dr. Paul Williams (antilordotic) or accompanying the flexion exercises with which his name is associated (Williams exercises), would be considered inappropriate today. They call for severe decrease in the lumbar lordosis, which is an attempt to reduce a swayback, the accentuation of lordosis which is considered a problem, but the loss of lordosis becomes a problem in itself, as it places the spine in an unnatural position and exerts undue force on the posterior longitudinal ligament, which is the vulnerable area for disc rupture under the influence of these forward flexed positions. So the best situation is a balance between these two extremes; that is, of a normal lordosis or a mild sway in the low back. So even though the Williams flexion exercises are by far the most commonly prescribed in doctors' offices, the consistent postures presented along with these exercises are understood to be inappropriate ("slouching"). In recent years, we would object to the flexion exercises as being "the" exercises, as the spine is designed to accomplish many functions through a significant variety of positions and limiting to these or only concentrating on a few would not accommodate the variety of actions required for activities of daily living or normal occupational use of the back.

More recently, the MacKenzie exercises have been promoted by many practitioners. These are actually part of a more comprehensive program and evaluation, based upon repetitive motion and the result of those repeated motions, and includes a set of exercises far beyond the extension exercises (Figure 9) that have become most familiar as they are distinctly different from the flexion exercises. Robin MacKenzie has popularized a program that would include the need to perform extension exercises, which brings the spine into a position of normal lordosis and theoretically would reverse an internal disc disruption or relieve pressure on a disc that is protruding toward the neural elements by producing a force to direct shifting of clumped disc material back toward the center of the nucleus pulposus and away from nerve roots. Many studies have been done showing that the extension exercises seem to have a higher rate of pain relief than the flexion exercises and certainly there will be patients who will benefit from either the flexion or the extension exercises and we should not limit ourselves to only one or the other of these types. Interestingly, the patient who has dehydrated discs and increased pressure on facet joints is likely to have stiff facets, and this situation is commonly seen by practitioners who note flexion and extension routinely on examination of their patients, particularly those with back pain, finding that the majority have limited extension while many are easily able to go into a full forward flexed position. It is unlikely that most individuals have any time during their day when they actually go into extension, although flexion is part of sitting and hence, extension would be expected to be restricted not only from facet disease and natural aging of the spine, but also from lack of ever stretching the spine into that position to retain normal nutrition of the disc and facet joints through motion, as we have discussed earlier.

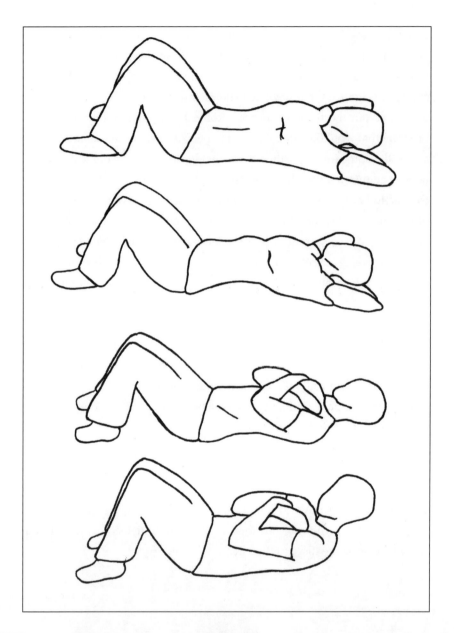

Figure 8

Stretching Exercises

Pelvic tilt, by alternately arching the back away from the floor while pressing the buttocks into the floor, will stretch the ligaments in the low back. Doing partial sit ups will exercise the abdominal muscles and hip/pelvic flexors.

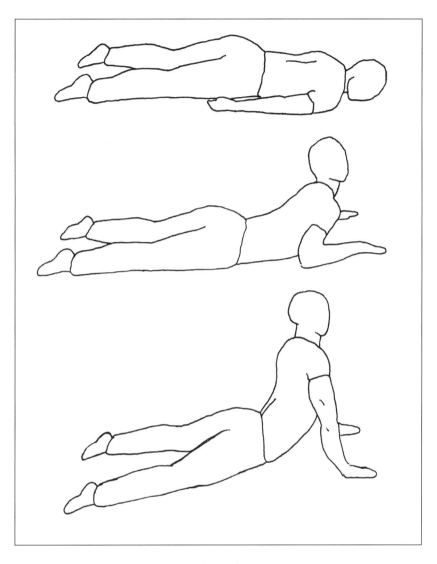

Figure 9

Extension exercises are performed by lying face down and initially relaxing in that posture. Progressing to pushing up to the elbows increases lumber extension and then gradually continuing up to the extended arms, sometimes facilitated by a belt holding the waist to the exercise table and across the pelvis to facilitate this exercise. These exercises are to stretch gradually, not to achieve a painful position and hold in that limit of extension for a prolonged period, but to come to the limit of the range of motion and gradually increase.

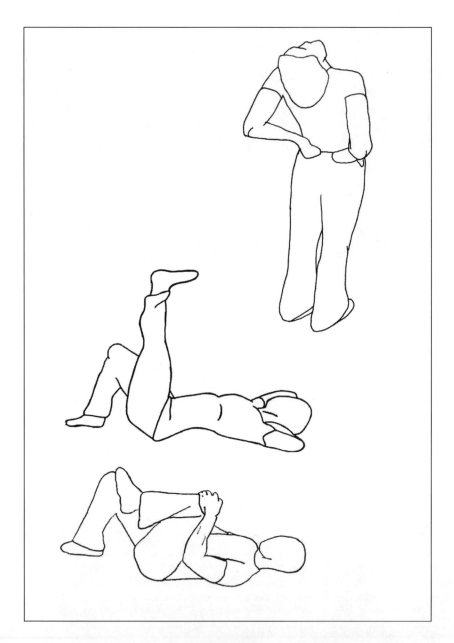

Figure 10

People who sit for prolonged periods are well advised to stand and do the illustrated extension exercise in place. Whenever we bend, the motion is primarily at the hip thus stretching the hamstrings is essential to maximize hip motion and minimize stress on the low back.

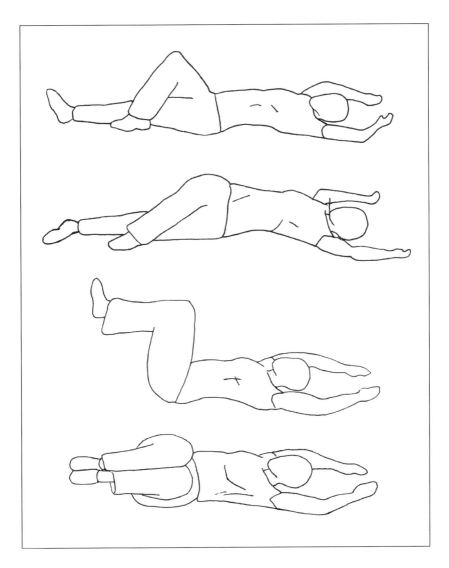

Figure 11

The orientation of the lumbar facet joints is vertical and allows flexion; rotation primarily occurs in the thoracic spine due to the orientation of those facet joints. Stretching increases this range of motion and allows the brain to select an optimum position of painless normal motion. Gentle stretching with rotation is appropriate; stretching should focus on trunk muscles particularly rotators, which have complex coordinated motions beyond our present scientific understanding.

STRETCHING

Stretching exercises take many forms, some of which should be familiar, as in Lamaze training or other areas. When we tighten muscles, following the tightening, we have the opportunity to release tension to a greater extent for relaxation, than if we just try to concentrate separately on relaxation. Many times we will have pain if we try to stretch muscles, particularly after we have had some injury or the onset of new pain. As a consequence, and almost solely with the low back, people are resistant to stretching because it hurts and they are afraid that it will cause more damage. If it was a stiff elbow, we would try to move the elbow without fear of further damage, but the mystery of the back means that we are intimidated and afraid to stretch the low back. Unfortunately, it may be necessary to do stretching and failure to stretch may prolong the pain. There is a threshold where the stretching will be just below the pain onset and this is where stretching is probably the most effective, although sometimes we would have to go up into the pain area above that threshold. When we need to exceed the pain threshold, this may require some supervision but generally muscles themselves have a variable length with varying tension, so it is not the muscle belly that needs the stretching, it is the tendon associated with that muscle and the fascia or the enveloping fibrous tissue over the muscle which may be tight. We need to stretch with a goal in mind, which is to achieve an increase in range of motion, which is necessary for recovery and to get back to normal. So, if we stretch and it exceeds the pain threshold, the suggestion would be just to stretch until there seems to be some increase in motion, not to cause excessive pain but to accept some pain if that happens. After the stretching exercises, the use of the muscles in any activities which warm up the muscles and cause blood to flow, should soften the fascia to assist in the stretching. This also can be accomplished with warm moist heat, a wet towel in the microwave for so-called modalities and physical therapy.

Clearly, if the muscles of the back are swollen, then the swelling may represent an impediment to the range of motion even without contracture or the tissues being too tight. Exercises in this case may be most helpful, not just to get back to normal range of motion, but also by the pressure of attempting normal range of motion to facilitate the exudation of the fluid—

to force out the fluid by going back to full range of motion. These may be done in bed and the first would be to lie flat, face down (prone) and to do extension exercises as the spine needs to go into extension; second, to do pelvic tilt or lying face up (supine) to flex the spine and finally to exercise the legs. This would be straight leg raising, which is hamstring stretch, and knee-to-chest exercises, which is using the abdominal muscles as well the quads. These exercises may not appeal to the heavy manual laborer, as they do not appear sufficiently strenuous and may seem like the doctor failed to recognize that they have a "real" problem. Nonetheless, these exercises that stretch the muscles of the back will resist the stiffening of the back and tightening of the fascia aligned with the muscles and should facilitate the resolution of swelling in the muscle. If there is a lot of swelling, which is blood or hemorrhage into the muscles from a muscle tear or muscle injury, then rest is necessary to some extent. First, significant pain is present; and second, the muscle itself is not being stretched and these fibers need to recover to some extent before we forcibly stretch them. Actually having hemorrhage into the muscles is an unusual situation and is not seen with the common lifting something at work and my back "gave out" or "I had pain in my back after I was doing this repetitive specific activity."

From the standpoint of the abdominal wall muscles (Figure 8), we often see after the laxity of the muscles in the abdomen from pregnancy or from other problems, that sit-ups are recommended. This clearly can be accomplished initially by isometric tensing of the muscles, as this is repetitively and gradually done over the course of several days, even for sore aching muscles. The isometric exercises can start to stretch and further exude some of the swelling in the tissues. Patients who have tight abdominal muscles would best lie flat on their stomach and after relaxing in this position may start some of the extension exercises (Figure 9) by pushing themselves up to the elbows or even up to the extended arms, not only stretching the anterior muscles but also stretching the joints of the facets in the posterior elements of the spine, which may be contracted from not having been in the extended position for a long time. It is interesting that an almost universal relief of tension is achieved by stretching into an extension position. Doing this in an exaggerated form may be therapeutic, but further exercise may also allow strengthening of these muscles.

Stretching is essential for stabilization of the pelvis as a platform for the low back muscles to work. Further, the hamstrings are specifically a potential problem if they are shortened or contracted. The range of motion of the hip is restricted by a tight hamstring. The actual movement in the back when we bend over is a small amount of the total motion: the majority of motion comes from the hips. If the hips are restricted, you put excessive strain on the low back in attempting to bend forward. Hence, stretching out the hamstrings (Fig 10) can prevent further injury, as well as be an important part of treatment.

As we have discussed previously, facet problems are frequent and may benefit from manipulation. To some extent, extension exercises as presented by MacKenzie in his book, *Treat Your Own Back,* and Robin MacKenzie, being a manipulative therapist from New Zealand (essentially a chiropractor from our standpoint), would suggest that to some extent these mobilization (Figure 11) exercises would reduce the need for manipulation, at least in that setting of patients treated in New Zealand. As back problems are not drastically different in nature, we might expect exercises that would isolate the facet joint, to provide a stretch force on that capsule, may be of some benefit. Beyond the extension mode, we would then introduce some element of rotation as a modified manipulation that may be performed, basically by rolling in bed with one leg over the side of the bed but the trunk left lying on the bed. This is somewhat similar to some positions during manipulation and we could at least call it soft-tissue mobilization, the necessary precursor to performing manipulation effectively and helpfully. Nonetheless, we are then performing an active exercise that would simulate the type of motion performed in manipulation, focusing on mobilizing or manipulating facet joint. As active involvement is part of this description, we would then be increasing our range of motion, which should result in the ability of the exerciser to achieve a wider range of postures without pain. Having done so actively, we would then be able to increase our activities and then, perhaps, do exercises more aggressively to rotate the low back and manipulate or at least mobilize the facet joints. The chiropractor may be helpful in starting out, if this is a particular component of the problem, but any active involvement of the patient will result in an appropriate response on the part of the back muscles and joint, not only to relieve the problem but perhaps to maintain range of motion, and prevent having the problem occur as frequently or being restricted by fear of recurrence of the pain.

STRENGTHENING

Strengthening exercises for the abdominal muscles are simply sit-ups and curls, but certainly more vigorous exercises can be performed with a rowing machine or other exercise equipment. Muscle strengthening for back extension would require not only raising the torso but also raising the legs (Figure 12) which should not only strengthen the spine extensors, but also the gluteus and hamstrings. Hip and thigh strengthening can be performed with a stationary bicycle or with wall slide exercises. Perhaps some of the best exercises are in the water, as aquatics allow not only flexibility through various positions, but resistance of the water, while relieving stress on the spine because of buoyancy, allows for strengthening of all the muscle groups . While we have described some exercises and provided some examples, general aerobic conditioning is an essential part of recovery. Basically, if an exercise allows a light sweat and elevates the heart rate to 140 or 150 beats a minute, then that exercise should increase air breathing or aerobic conditioning. In general, the heart rate maximum is roughly 220 minus age, that maximum can be multiplied times some factor, such as eighty percent, which then becomes the desired maximum achieved heart rate during exercise. The eighty percent will provide a level of safety below the maximum. While we do strengthening exercises, we should be causing blood to flow into those muscles and secondarily increasing our cardiovascular capabilities.

When we consider strengthening, we should realize that the hamstrings and gluteal muscles in the legs have five times the bulk and, hence, with roughly equivalent strength per bulk, five times the strength of the lumbar muscles. It is evident that these muscles are active and part of motions to stabilize the spine and, thus, need to be strengthened to stabilize the pelvis. If the pelvis is stable, the muscles of the spine can operate more efficiently and painlessly. It is, therefore, reasonable to start with lower extremity muscle strengthening (Figure 12) and rehabilitation prior to using back machines and trying to strengthen back muscles directly, which may remain painful

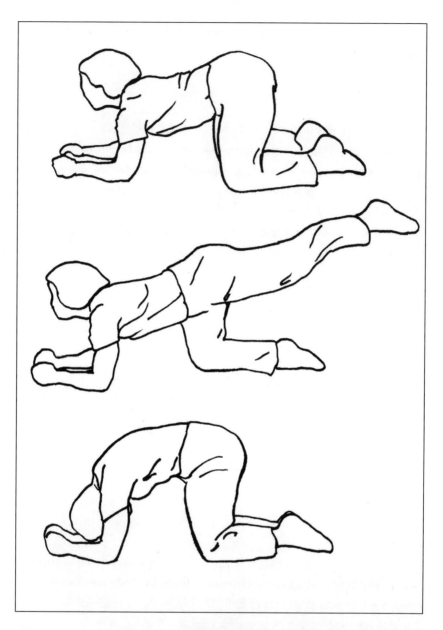

Figure 12

The cat back exercise involves stretching the spine ligaments and muscles, but also strengthens the muscles. Specifically the hamstrings are strengthened when the leg is elevated and extended behind a person.

after the injury and need to have the lower extremity muscles first rehabilitated. This is commonly referred to as pelvic stabilization, with physical therapy plans written by the therapist as part of evaluating of the patient, recommended for the physician's signature as a treatment plan.

Below this level of eighty percent of the maximum achievable heart rate, we should be achieving a light sweat and the conditioning exercises should continue to strengthen muscles but also to improve our general cardiovascular conditioning. As we are able to do more and more exercise, we should progress slowly on an approximately weekly basis, as the interval for increasing the number of repetitions or weights used in the exercises. The goal is to try to keep the heart rate at the same elevated level and to maintain it, so we have a stable amount of stress on the cardiovascular system which really has an increase of the amount of work capability as we become stronger and healthier. This can be with a rowing machine, back and hip or knee exercise machines, or just with walking or swimming. Exercises have been described as stabilizing for the spine and some of these are intended specifically to strengthen the erector spinae in the back, and then the stabilizing of the pelvic girdle (gluteal and hamstrings). It should be noted, as the disc dehydrates, that there is a lack of stability and an increase in the motion that occurs. This increase in motion can pull on soft tissues with pain fibers and result in low back pain. With time, this may lead to degenerative spurs and stiffening of the spine, both by the spurs and collagenization or scarring of the disc, but the concept of strengthening for stabilization is appropriate and should be emphasized. Having discussed stretching exercises and strengthening or now stabilizing exercises, we will reserve the rehabilitation or reconditioning exercises for a later discussion of work hardening and endurance, as returning to work is usually a forty-hour-a-week situation, as opposed to a few hours in physical therapy. Further, these exercises are usually performed with specific equipment, making a simulation of the job, so that it is not realistic on your own but becomes considerably more specific than the exercises discussed thus far.

Having attempted to demystify the issue of exercises, I am sure that the generalizations used to make the point that exercises are not magical or complicated, will leave some readers with a curiosity about specific examples. Even if I went into much greater detail and a much longer description of specific exercises, the role of the physical therapist in supervising and, particularly, in reassuring the patient that the exercises were performed correctly, would certainly remain a medically necessary and significant benefit. However, I would suggest that the role of the therapist should be considered interventional rather than maintenance. It should not only supervise but reassure the patient that the exercises are done properly. After a patient has been evaluated and become practiced in doing specific exercises, and after the therapist has evaluated those exercises and determines that they are appropriate and correctly performed, the next step should logically be that the therapist will teach the patient how to proceed and continue on his own. It is not only expensive to perpetuate supervised therapy, but the patient needs to be empowered to treat his own back. Workers need to understand body mechanics and not do unsafe movements and cause injury. They also need to know how to respond to incidental minor aggravations of daily living. It has been interesting to me, observing that recovery after extensive back surgery is quite prolonged, that patients who come back five to ten years later say that everything is fine but wow did they take a long time! My experience has been that some cases of back problems do far better with a trainer than with a therapist because the time constraints upon a trainer to get somebody back for next season are different in the basic mindset of the training professional from the therapist who is trying to get somebody back to work to save income and to get them as quickly as possible back to normal. Acute intervention is appropriate and necessary; however, backs are so slow that it is almost a different problem. It is often semi-acute, or in many cases, clearly a chronic problem. If this is realized, the patient is better treated; some patients did far better with a trainer.

Prior to discussing any of the specific exercises, there are two notes that should be made. First, if patients do hamstring stretching and notice that as the leg is raised with the knee straight and there is a shooting electric shock down the leg, this is sciatica or possibly the radiculopathy of a nerve irritated by a ruptured disc. This occurs in less than two percent of patients who are newly complaining of low back pain in the family practice setting; but when it does occur, it is an indication for imaging studies (CT scan, preferably MRI). The patient who has vague pain down the leg may have irritation of facet joints and muscle problems, but specifically raising the leg

with the knee straight and having shooting pain down the leg, not count-
ing pain noticed in the back from that maneuver, should be referred to a
physician and not embark on any exercises. Secondly, patients who come
back into extension and have weakness in their legs, particularly patients in
their sixties or older and those who walk progressively forward flexed as
they walk any short distance, may have spinal stenosis, and these patients
may benefit from extension exercises to free up arthritic facet joints. On
occasions when they have weakness, numbness, or pain to the legs, specific therapy and even surgical intervention may be required. Finally, as an
overall comment, any patients who have worse pain at rest or at night, have
the risk of having a tumor or an infection and these patients should
promptly see a physician for appropriate X rays and other evaluation to
reassure them regarding the most serious, though rare, problems which
may distinguish themselves from other back pain by this characteristic;
namely, if as a patient lies in bed there is often an engorgement of pelvic
veins and this will increase pressure in a tumor, causing worse pain at bed
rest. Further, these are not mechanical pains, as the pressure from an infection or from a tumor builds up regardless of whether we are doing anything; and, hence, at night even without further activity of the day to wors-
en degenerated disc or arthritic facet joints, these patients will have worsening pain. These symptoms, even without a fever, call for an urgent examination by the physician.

MEDICATIONS

An oversimplified but perhaps realistic appraisal of treatments offered
for low back pain short of surgery is that they are intended to allow inflammation to resolve. As we see in acute injury, there may be muscle spasm
that may be relatively prominent. In those cases, we not only recommend
lying in bed to relieve the spasm, but also modalities such as ice or heat, and
then eventually some exercises; and just as we bring the toes up to tighten
the gastrocnemius and resist a muscle cramp in the calf, we may find good
relaxation of muscle spasm by resisting gently and then allowing the muscle to fatigue and release the spasm. Most effective on muscle spasms are
ice treatments but chronic spasms benefit from heat. Beyond the physical

modalities that are customarily attempted by Mom for injured children, the adult is unable to continue customary activities and wants a quick fix, so presents to the doctor. When people present to the emergency room, they expect to have a powerful medication prescribed and often muscle relaxants are used for the acute episode. Unfortunately, muscle relaxants are then commonly abused later when muscle spasm is no longer present. For an initial episode, the muscle relaxants, may be effective, but when the spasms have resolved, the relaxants are no longer appropriate. My preference is to avoid the use of muscle relaxants, if possible, particularly after about two weeks, since all of them basically seem to have a more central effect of sedating the patient than selectively to relax the muscles. There are cases of degenerative changes, arthritic stimulation of inflammation, and other reasons for recurring muscle spasms on an episodic basis for which muscle relaxants would be helpful, but these are the exception rather than the rule.

Most patients have some form of inflammation, and as such it would be appropriate to use an anti-inflammatory. Obviously, aspirin or the variations on Motrin and Alleve, which are also over the counter, can be available easily to the patient and may have a beneficial effect. Prescription anti-inflammatories, often longer acting, are more convenient to take on a regular basis, or more easily achieve a full therapeutic anti-inflammatory dose with fewer pills than taking the over- the- counter dose of aspirin or Motrin. Unfortunately, most acute injuries are treated with a narcotic such as codeine and a muscle relaxant. The muscle relaxant is of short duration benefit, if any, and shortly becomes a potential problem; and the narcotic is inappropriate for any chronic problem. Initially, the problem is acute; but when the patient experiences some relief from the medication and when they have increased pain on withdrawal of the narcotic, it is easy to get involved in a chronic situation where habituating narcotics have been used or are being requested for at least some relief of the pain.

The ideal reliever of inflammation is the steroid type medication, and tapering doses of steroids are often used for acute injuries. These are medications like prednisone or forms of cortisone, a naturally occurring hormone which is released under conditions of stress. The medical forms are synthesized artificially to increase the anti-inflammatory effect, while diminishing the other effects on blood sugar and salt regulation in the body. Inflammation, for example, from extensive poison ivy, that is, contact dermatitis, or reaction to a bee sting or other acute reactions, may be a cause for the use of oral steroids, that is, systemic or through the whole body. Inflammation of the eye which could cause corneal scarring and loss of sight may certainly require a short-term use of steroids, particularly topically in the eye. Pain in the back, particularly which seems to have radiation down the leg and irritation of a nerve root, may benefit from a short pulse of high-dose steroids tapering off over about a week to ten days' time. All of the anti-inflammatory drugs other than steroids themselves are actually called nonsteroidal anti-inflammatories and are less effective, but both the steroids and the nonsteroidal basically are distributed to the entire body and as such, a higher dose has to be used than would be locally, for example, by injection.

The key concern is that the physician is not bullied into using stronger medicine by the patient who feels, because of the pain, the need for an immediate amelioration or relief of the problem. Certainly there is controversy about sending athletes back into the game pumped up with steroids. We know on a body building or other muscle-training level, that steroids can enhance performance but have serious, even lethal effects. As a professional, the physician has to understand that the demand or the need for the patient to have immediate results may be an economic or a psychological problem rather than a physical demand. Penicillin will cure a strep throat in a few days, so we advise rest, fluids, and aspirin to help for those few days. People who demand an immediate gratifying result are common, and I do not mean to be critical of them since this reaction flows from the anxiety which is common surrounding back injuries and back problems. It is nonetheless the professional's responsibility to take the long view and recognize, having X rays to show that it is not cancer or infection or fracture, but to reassuringly proceed along a reasonable course, recognizing that even steroids, although beneficial in the short term, have hazards that are not insignificant; and if the inflammation is resolved, then the rate of resolution may not merit those hazards.

In addition to anti-inflammatory medications, chronic pain is often associated with muscle tightness, joint stiffness, and a sleep disorder as previously described under the section on fibrositis. We have in mind a classical concept of pain, where an ancient Chinese artwork shows a toe in the fire, a line drawing a signal up to the brain causing withdrawal reflex and pulling the toe out of the fire because it hurts. We are, of course, aware that the brain communicates to the spinal cord to the hands and feet and the hands feel things, which are sensory nerves going up to the brain, and in response, the muscles function under our voluntary control by motor nerves. Unfortunately, pain is not that simple. Describing pain in terms of intensity or severity is like seeing a black-and-white universe in two dimensions. Some pain in our hands and feet may be a result, not of a pinched nerve from a disc problem, but from a sick nerve, such as a diabetic neuropathy in which the nerves are damaged because of poor control of our blood sugar; or similarly, lead toxicity or mercury poisoning can cause damage to nerves.

Further, there is pain commonly associated with fibrositis or which is frequently seen in chronic pain syndromes, which we refer to as sympathetically mediated. This type of pain is associated with the sympathetic system, or the involuntary nervous system. To illustrate, we know that if we are scared because a car pulled out in front of us with short notice and we hit the brakes hard to avoid a collision, we feel flushed or red in the face, our heart beats fast, it may skip a few beats. If we have an interview under hostile circumstances, we may have sweaty palms from nervousness as well as a dry mouth and it is difficult to form our words under stress. These changes in our physical status, heart rate and so forth are from the response of the sympathetic nervous system to our fear. We are not consciously aware of control of our body functions, such as sweating, the pilomotor function which makes our hair stand up, or goose bumps; but obviously there are involuntary or unconscious systems working, causing our blood pressure to increase under stress and our heart rate to miss beats or go faster when we are startled. A significant injury, particularly with severe soft-tissue swelling, such as a crush injury, is often associated with changes in the involuntary nervous system. These may be referred to as dysfunction or dystrophy of the sympathetic system, a reflex sympathetic dystrophy. That is part of what has been called in more recent times a complex regional pain syndrome: for example, there may be a severe reflex pain in the hand or the foot, even though the swelling has to a significant extent, or perhaps even completely, resolved. The reflexive pain of the reflex sympathetic dystrophy, or a causalgia or a "Sudek Atrophy," has been in the past poorly recognized or denied; in the present it is being studied aggressively and will remain relatively under recognized or under diagnosed in medical treatment. Please allow some analogies to illustrate these sympathetic systems.

If a person goes outdoors and waits at the bus stop on a cold day, the skin temperature of that person will go from a comfortable warm level while indoors, to a much cooler level when they are outdoors in the elements. That decrease in skin temperature will cause an increased difference between the skin temperature and the deeper body tissue's temperature, effectively creating an insulation barrier and reducing the loss of heat. This is by arteries and veins which are superficial, basically shunting or redirecting the blood deeper and restricting the amount of blood that flows superficially. With less superficial blood flow to have that blood cooled and be taken back to the heart and the core, and thus need to be reheated metabolically, a person would lose less heat by having the involuntary nervous system allow the superficial skin temperature to decrease. Unfortunately, patients who have this sympathetic or involuntary system stuck in the off or on position may have excess swelling, may feel significant pain without identifiable cause in terms of voluntary nerves, that is, sensory or motor. This type of pain has a complex origin and requires extensive treatment. However, there may be an element that involves a lot of less severe injuries, so some of the medications used may seem to be inappropriate or not specific and often are denied by the insurance carriers out of cost concerns and the explanations are unconvincing to those who refuse to be convinced and difficult for those who are interested.

Patients who have vascular insufficiency or atherosclerosis may have pain in their extremities, and one of the treatments that is done to try to increase the blood flow (prior, in a sense, to rotorooting the pipes surgically) is for the sympathetic nerves that control the blood vessels to be destroyed or cut so that the system is left on. This leads to a warmer, more vascular extremity as all the peripheral circuits are now open which may reduce some pain. This is also done for patients who have had a severely swollen extremity, that continues to be painful even though X rays have shown no fracture and the swelling has started to recede and time has passed so the usual expectation would be of benefit. Unfortunately, the same effect of closing off blood vessels at the bus stop to increase insulation occurs when people light a cigarette. The vasoconstriction is beneficial in terms of heat loss, so most people who smoke, light a cigarette when they are out in the cold. But they also counteract the beneficial effect that might be had for their circulation, not only in the heart but also in the extremities as well as to the brain and kidneys. In fact, three cigarettes a day will decrease the oxygen tension in one's intervertebral discs to less than half. So, even though we know coughing may cause an increase in back pain in people with damaged discs and smokers clearly cough more often and more deeply, we have other reasons to suspect the severe deterioration of patients' discs who smoke. Further, when we try to treat patients who have pain from a medical standpoint or with medications, the results may be negated and totally ineffective when patients continue to smoke.

Patients who have difficulty sleeping are often given a low dose anti-depressant for chronic pain and stiff muscles not, specifically, because of depression and not in a dose sufficient for depression, although chronic pain is depressing, but to counteract the involuntary nervous system effects which perpetuate and accentuate pain. Some people feel a moderation or diminution of the severity of their pain with these medications. So, in a comprehensive rehabilitation approach, when they are used, people sometimes reject them out of hand because they say, "I really got hurt at work and it's not just all in my head. I am not depressed." In fact, the doctor realizes that the longstanding nature of the pain or, specifically, some of the components that are described as burning or "my feet feel cold" are typical for sympathetically medicated pain that might benefit from specific medications. Some of these would include vasodilators, so Procardia may be used to open blood vessels in the sense that a sympathetic block helps patients who have persistent swelling and pain after a crush injury. These medications are quite widely used but often with poor compliance because the patient does not understand the motivation as described above. When used infrequently, and without an understanding that these are truly to moderate pain rather than because the doctor believes a patient is faking, they can be of significant benefit.

Injections

The use of injected steroids or numbing medicines (anesthetics) for various problems has been well established. Inflamed joints may be quieted with pain relief and function restored by intra-articular or intrabursal injection of long-acting forms of steroids. Similarly, injections have been used in the spine with various intentions. First, injections of local anesthetics as well as corticosteroids may have a diagnostic role in establishing that the pain is originating from the spine and radiating distantly, and second, help in selective localization. Next, the corticosteroid is in a slowly dissolving form, such that it is effective in relieving the inflammation; and, thus, the pain for a prolonged interval may demonstrate that there is a significant inflammatory component, rather than the otherwise assumed mechanical etiology. If it returns, then the underlying pathology, rather than some recent overuse or sprain is then at fault.

From a teleological standpoint, or basically: if it's there, there must have been a reason; the inflammation may have some role in healing and certainly the inflammation of the lining of a joint, the synovium, has a role in digesting the wear products from the joint surfaces. While this digestion process is painful and causes fluid or joint swelling or joint effusion, it can be diminished with steroids but with some toxicity to the articular surfaces. This toxicity in terms of interfering with the inflammatory response or the early part of the healing reaction of the body would naturally cause concern if repeatedly done in muscles or around ligaments and tendons on an excessive basis. Customary practice includes occasional injections with significant separating intervals and the recognition that surgical synovectomy in large joints or other means would be appropriate after repetition becomes addiction.

The expectation that the injection will have a prolonged benefit in terms of changing the underlying structure is unrealistic, as the injections are basically anti-inflammatories. When inflammation presents as an episodic problem and not chronic or arthritic, then recovery may in some cases be expected. Subsequent exercise and good fitness are essential as a coupled treatment to go along with the injection. So, even if the injection cannot improve the situation by building up or strengthening the underlying structure, if the relief of pain allowed by the injected medication promotes exercise and the patient is motivated to become actively involved in a rehabilitation program, then recovery in an overall meaningful sense can be accomplished. Unfortunately, many cases who have an increase in swelling or symptoms in the knee, elbow, or even the spine may initially respond to steroids, but the progression of the arthritic disease or degeneration may result in the appearance that the steroid is no longer effective. Effectiveness of the steroid remains but it is not adequate to resolve all problems. When there is structural damage, the structural damage is not going to be corrected by the medication, which is only relieving the inflammation.

The therapeutic role of injection remains somewhat controversial and probably is not relevant without some degeneration. Although anesthetic agents that are injected ease the pain of the injection, they also may reset the sympathetic system, to some extent; and this may be helpful as described previously for sympathetic overdrive or sympathetic dystrophy; however, single injections are not always useful and a therapeutic series of injections is often required. In the presence of degeneration, then the arthritic changes may benefit from the diminution of inflammation as described above and this may result in increased function and restoration of muscle tone and joint flexibility. However, if there is a simple disc herniation, which is a mechanical force on a nerve root and sciatica, then surgery will not be prevented, only delayed by steroid injection. This would particularly be the deep injection, usually by an anesthesiologist, into the epidural space. (Figure 13) that is, the space around the nerve roots but not into the sac that contains those nerve roots and the spinal fluid. A block that will relieve some pain but not have full elimination of muscular activity, such as a saddle block is also used obstetrically. The epidural is with a steroid for inflammation, unlike the short-acting anesthetic used for delivery in obstetrics.

While an injury or overactivity may cause inflammation interfering with activity and not resolve despite rest or inactivity, the steroid may allow resolution of the situation and recovery if appropriately rehabilitated following the injection: that is, not immediately but definitely following with some exercises to increase joint range of motion and muscle tone and decrease adhesions or scarring, not presuming that the problem is resolved and automatically will care for itself. If injections are into a trigger point, or as we discussed with fibrositis, a knot in the muscle that is so painful that the patient has trouble combing his or her hair or doing activities of daily living, the injection may allow resumption of activities and then gradual exercise so that the muscles may be relaxed by having been tensed and exercised, thus leading to resumption of activity.

If a joint is quite swollen, then an injection along with medication of the anti-inflammatory type may allow resumption of activity and satisfactory function. This, however, does not preclude either the progression of the disease or the chronic desire on the part of the patient for injections. As such, the injections form a poor routine to dose unlike medication, as they need to be spaced by weeks or months rather than hours like pills, and further, they require a needle to inject locally a large amount of medication so that it is not distributed all over the entire body as are oral medications. Nonetheless, the body's natural ability to produce natural steroid hormones may be suppressed by repeated chronic steroid injections; and, hence, this component occasionally has to be checked.

Acupuncture and various other novel injection techniques, such as sclerotherapy for loose painful ligaments or also prolotherapy, have been used and have varying successes in individual cases. No dramatic generally applicable results are evident from these various treatments. In a field that involves considerable competition among practitioners for patients and a great diversity of treatments with promotion of many- good results cannot be hidden and if reported by any practitioner, will subsequently easily be duplicated by many others. Albeit grateful for occasional successes, these many alternative treatments have to be noted as having a limited role overall and a certain lack of optimism when the promoters of any particular technique have to tout an individual practitioner's skill in performing the technique as essential for the success quoted. It then almost becomes a matter where from a critical standpoint the success may be partly that of the patient being convinced by this charismatic practitioner, or a placebo effect, in addition to whatever therapeutic merit the treatment may have. If the

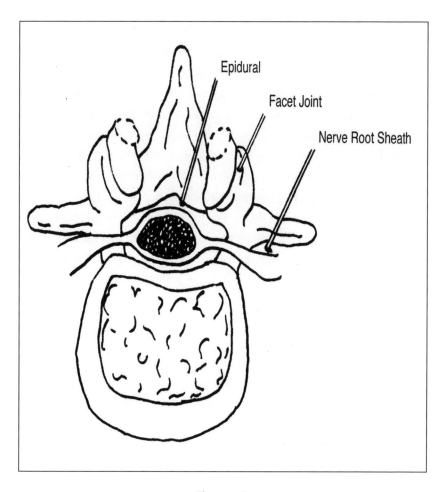

Epidural

Facet Joint

Nerve Root Sheath

Figure 13

Injections around the sac (dura), which contains the nerves, are epidural injections. As the facet joint may be irritated and inflamed, some injections are directly into the facet joint. Some practitioners will inject medication along the nerve root sheath after exit from the spinal column: when the needle causes radiating pain down the leg to indicate that it is at the point of the nerve root, then in this vicinity, the medication is injected. Injections are also in that order of commonness: most common the epidural, next most common the facet injection, and then nerve root sheath injections, less common.

treatment is not readily reproduced and equally satisfactory in result by other practitioners, then a rational scientific basis for its success will be exceedingly hard to establish.

DRUGS AND DETOX

As many of these patients have had or will have pain for extended periods, the effects of chronic pain, the implications of which we will discuss in the next chapter, result in considerable suffering. These severe effects cause the patient to naturally request relief and, particularly, pain medication for the problem. When anti-inflammatories fail to relieve the pain, stronger medication is requested and this seems humanely to be the physician's only choice. If narcotics are prescribed, a chronic problem is a contraindication to a narcotic by its very nature. That is, longer use will have diminishingly smaller benefit from a narcotic (tolerance) but addiction becomes a risk and complicating problem secondary to the back pain. This problem may require treatment in and of itself and certainly is not a good sign as the patient has become drug dependent and the side effects of narcotics include constipation, secondary depression, irritability as well as widely recognized drug-seeking behavior: manipulation, paranoia, and distress.

We will discuss in the next chapter acute and chronic pain from a more general sense, but, certainly, chronic pain is not appropriately first treated with a short-term solution like narcotics. For this reason, many centers first may have to allow the patient sufficient activities and instruction in behavioral modification so that they can wean themselves from the narcotics. Patients react against psychological treatment because the feeling is that they have been abandoned and not believed and that the doctor feels it is all in their head. Yet, no one doubts the doctor's diagnosis when they are overweight, as the scales don't lie (although we usually think they are exaggerating some); and, yet, in that case, even nonmedical programs emphasize behavioral control. The NIH has developed a program to recommend how physicians should discuss smoking with their patients as an effective means of helping some quit this unhealthy habit. A lot of effort has gone into behavioral modification and the specific things to say and emphasize that should be effective. Clearly patients who have been on narcotics for a significant period of time need to have at least as much psychological support and alternate activities to turn to, rather than the drugs, when they are experiencing pain. Psychological support, for quitting smoking or dieting and behavioral modification, is a keystone of this treatment, but not pragmatically available unless part of a comprehensive rehabilitation program as we will discuss.

Because there genuinely is pain, one of the important matters may be first to put the patient on long-acting narcotics such as oxycontin, a patch, methadone or even steroid injections that may last for many weeks as a basis of distracting from the medications that are short term and, hence, quick relief, but really support their denial rather than recovery. That is, if when you have pain you take a pill for relief, then that becomes a conditioned reflex and any efforts to stop the pills requires the elimination of the pain rather than improvement, or pills are taken on the same schedule. When pain first has to be eliminated as a precondition to get off drugs, then it will never happen, as pains are gradually improved rather than being immediately eliminated in the real world (staircase effect, not sudden cure).

While the detoxification programs are not ideal for all patients, some by being cooperative and actively involved in the program, recognize their need to be involved and instructed in behavioral techniques, and these patients, particularly, take advantage of the opportunity. In many cases, the difficult problem of chronic pain is intertwined with the overall situation that has resulted in lack of self esteem, frustration, and defeat in financial recovery or return to productivity. As we will discuss in the next chapter, the problem of chronic pain needs to be recognized. If acute pain is not differentiated from chronic pain, as we will discuss in the next chapter, any attempts to treat the patient on an acute pathophysiologic basis, as if pain indicates ongoing tissue damage or injury rather than a mechanical irritation and subsequent pain from activities, will be unsuccessful and only perpetuate the chronic pain disease. As we attempt to provide a lay description of chronic pain that is understandable to the reader, the point that should be emphasized is that a program which fails to recognize chronic pain which does not have resources necessary to deal with such a problem including psychological support (genuinely provided—not as an afterthought or thrown in to satisfy criteria for a complete program), may result in a patient failure where the patient may have succeeded in a bona fide program.

SURGERY

Surgical indications start with the failure of nonsurgical care. Of course, it is essential that nonsurgical care be maximally offered in a way in which any possible result is achieved, ensuring that relief could not have occurred without surgery or that the surgical procedure was a necessity. Clearly, the nonsurgical techniques and methods are at least theoretically reducing inflammation from an acute injury. When there is a chronic injury such as arthritis, anti-inflammatory medications, injections or exercise may be of benefit but are not curative. As such, treatments which may permanently restore a person with back trouble to productivity would include work restrictions. This may not be a full recovery, but it is a change from disability to productivity with partial impairment. The use of an assistant at work or of modifications of the tasks done at work are also appropriate considerations which need to be fully exhausted before some surgeries are considered and are a primary part of the nonsurgical care.

When the patient has sciatica, a gratifying result is obtained when pressure is removed from a nerve root, such as in surgical laminectomy or discectomy. These procedures have been refined to a high level and can reliably be done with minimal postoperative convalescence and are to be recommended highly in cases that have the appropriate indications. It is, however, not expected that good results will automatically follow an excellent procedure when the need or the appropriateness of that procedure is questionable. This is the reason we have specifically discussed the indications; the pathology encountered, in hopes that some concept of the fact that a bulging disc does not need an operation, in the same sense that a herniated disc would indicate the possible need for surgery. Further, if a bulging disc is not pressing significantly on a nerve, then we can certainly expect, even in the most severe pain reports, that when there is a small nerve compromise from a bulging disc or a relatively small herniation, that there will only be a small benefit from relieving this small pressure on the nerves. This is obvious from the way I have described the situation, but it seems in most cases that the excellent results from a large disc herniation being operated are assumed to translate to an individual patient's case, as that patient is convinced that the pain is so severe that there must be a severe herniation; and, therefore, the surgical indications must certainly be appropriately met despite the surgeon's doubts. Although it seems a bit incredible, often there is a significant stress on the surgeon to "just try" the operation to see if it will help. This may seem a reasonable reaction on the part of the patient who is in pain and disabled and certainly has parallels with things I have asked my mechanic to do in my car when I was concerned about reliability and some components that seem to be working okay but not reliable or assured of longevity. Certainly we should at least have a reaction on the part of the physician, of delay in the consideration of an operative procedure whenever there is any improvement in the patient's symptoms or capabilities. While a relief of some of the swelling or a resolution of edema may occur over a period of time, waiting may be a significant part of evaluating the adequacy of non-surgical care before we consider doing an operation.

Generally, operating on scar is a fool's errand, as further surgery causes more scarring and there may be initial benefit, but it does not produce long-lasting relief of back problems. Patients who have had an operation may have a new disc herniation and this is a convenient explanation for the surgeon whose result has initially been good but then became inadequate or a failure, and hence the second operation may be considered. The results of second operations are diminishingly successful; and, unfortunately, removing a disc in a case where previous discs have been removed and now further disc material reappears, calls for an exceedingly cautious attitude. Particularly, if the herniation continues to reoccur, then we may be dealing with segmental instability, and need to recommend that rather than just the simple operation of removing a disc, surgical arthrodesis or a fusion is necessary. This is a major undertaking and should be only after prolonged conservative care to determine the necessity, but should be sooner than four or five unsuccessful disc operations. Early recognition of the true disease as being total structural incompetence of the disc rather than a portion of the disc rupturing and causing sciatica, particularly when there is a significant component of back pain rather than just the leg pain, is an essential part of the evaluation of the patient.

Patients who have an unstable disc may have back pain without significant radiculopathy or significant compression of nerves on their imaging studies, such as MRI. Patients who have had multiple disc operations need either to accept their disability at some point, or, perhaps, accept the inadequacy of a microdiscectomy or laminectomy type operation for their problem. If the disc is unstable and does not support the vertebra, taking a small portion of that disc away will not enhance its stability and may weaken or further destabilize that disc. If the problem is back pain, the radiating sciatica type pain from compression which responds well to a microdiscectomy or removing disc material from the nerve has no role in effecting the back pain. Patients with symptomatic spondylolisthesis have loss of bony support and need a fusion and in the long run do extremely well. Patients who have had multiple previous surgeries have often had relief of some of their leg pain but have continued back pain or in most cases worse back pain. This back pain may be disabling and it may be impossible to limit activities on the job or to do activities of daily living. These are cases which may be candidates for a fusion operation; that is, stabilizing the bad disc by interposing bony support where muscular strengthening has not adequately relieved the pain.

WORK HARDENING

Physical therapy and exercise is required for muscles to regain their tone and endurance, and this can effectively be accomplished by exercise machines or programs directed, monitored, and supervised by physical therapists or trainers. As we consider these programs and incorporate occupational therapists to modify for activities of daily living and provide accomodation rather than expectation of cure, the patient may remain productive and resume daily activities without a recurrence of the pain and disability. We then have a program that is more comprehensive and effective than just the exercise machines that consider the patients' progress on a strictly physical basis. We really have a different type of treatment, as most physical therapy facilities have limited space to accommodate patients for more than a treatment. When patients are expected to work for two hours and then later for four, and then progressively longer times for part of the day, they cannot be accommodated in physical therapy. As such, the work hardening programs are different in nature and often in location. Unfortunately, a physical therapy department with additional space and some newly acquired exercise machines is not a full work-hardening program.

Often in circumstances where work hardening is appropriate, simulation of a patient's job will allow the patient to do the lifting, shoveling, or other material manipulation that is much like what they would do on the job. If they are able to progress in lifting objects similar to their work materials, then as they perform those jobs under supervision with instruction in terms of body mechanics and technique, they can develop increased endurance and, hence, their early ability to return to work.

As patients progress, some pain may occur; and for this, modalities may occasionally be resorted to, but not on an extensive basis, as it represents a failure of the exercises for rehabilitation. Further, it can be a behavioral problem, since the patient should have progressed beyond the rest and inflammation stage, and, particularly, if narcotic medication is resumed. In such cases, it is important to gauge improvement by serial functional capacities evaluation or a lift test or any other means to evaluate whether the patient from week to week is able to perform more activities than previously. If there comes a point when the patient's ability to lift or perform physical functions is unimproved from previous weeks, then a plateauing should be documented; and as such, the program has essentially completed its task of maximal medical improvement, following which vocational rehabilitation or light duty work needs to be obtained.

When a patient has relief with exercise, it is necessary that the exercise progress to harden the patient or build endurance. In some cases, we will have a failure of the work hardening program in that the patient is not able to tolerate the increased effort or increased load because of the recurrence of pain or the increase in their pain. When there is increased pain on a particular task or exercise and this is needed to return the patient to work full time, or an increased variety of postures such as sitting alternating with standing and so forth are necessary to accommodate situations that arise on the job, we may come to an artificial stalemate where we are unable to return the patient to his previous position since, for example, light duty is not made available and retraining is not authorized. This situation may be understandable for a small company, but also occurs in other cases because of union rules. The practitioner's need at this point is to recognize that the patient cannot progress and not to take it personally, but to admit defeat and discontinue the program. To certify that the patient is able to return to work when the program is no longer able to help increase the batting average of that particular program and promote future business or referrals from the insurance company may lead in some cases to short-term return to work. In most cases, these patients will not continue on the job but will seek legal redress, resulting in depositions and legal action, eventually receiving disability benefits after a protracted battle and probably castigation of the employee for not being interested in working or trying hard enough, but never on the employer.

Patients often articulate a sincere desire to go back to their previous occupations, and while this makes us optimistic that they have a desire and should continue the programs, we may need on occasion to accept this as denial on the part of the patient and recognize that psychological or other job stress or job dysfunction factors need to be brought in, particularly if the patient ceases to progress in specific areas that create an inability to return to his previous job. The problem that we are dealing with is disability, the patient's inability to return to work. As such, the physical capabilities and the physical injury are an integral part, but the treatment is to return the patient to productivity, not to continue trying to return each patient to his original occupation as if on warranty, believing that modern medicine can cure any problem. Many patients will still have residual pain and they will be relatively comfortable when they are doing nothing, that is, not returning to work; but, they will be best off when the likelihood of their return to their previous occupation is recognized as minimal early in the treatment rather than after prolonged sequences of attempted work hardening. Without a vocational counselor, a lot of unfulfilling efforts have been expended for patients who just can't return to that job and that immediate supervisor, but the patients are unwilling to admit that it is really because they feel they were unfairly or inappropriately treated rather than injured.

FUNCTIONAL RESTORATION

A particularly successful and helpful program is described as the functional restoration program. This program is essentially work hardening with integration of psychological support based upon specific principles. The main underlying principle is that a patient may be able to increase her functional capacity without a commensurate increase in pain. That is, if the patient lifts twice as much but does not have twice as much pain, only slightly more, then as the patient continues increasing her activity, she has less pain than she previously did. In a sense, work hardening always involves some progression, but when the progression is by objective measures (more weight or more resistance on an exercise machine) rather than limited by the subjective experience of pain by the patient, progress can be made even with some pain and with the eventual result of pain reduction. This concept seems too easy to be true, or getting something for nothing. From a physiologic standpoint, we would assert that the increased exercise of the muscles allows better circulation, better nourishment, and better function of the whole back as a unit. As we progress, we also are uplifted in our hope and optimism and even our prospect of return to work and our previous enjoyment of our life and activities. Psychological support is an important part of such a program, emphasizing on-the-spot behavioral treatment of pain and emphasizing goal setting rather than inactivity to relieve acute inflammation. Incomplete versions of such a program (often copied, never duplicated) did not have results as good, and we need to have careful attention to function rather than pain with a specific behavioral modification program to expect the reported eighty-eight percent return to work.

One of the other important specialties is that of a vocational counselor. When a patient is unable to return to her job, either because of stress on the job, physical impairment, or a multitude of other reasonings, we need to retrain the patient along lines within her functional capacities. The functional capacities assessment is often sent to the physician by the insurance carrier who is seeking completion of the form by the physician subjectively, who is unable to complete it objectively without equipment, but in hopes that the physician will be bullied into filling it out while they threaten the patient with loss of income. If it is your doctor's fault that you can't get your compensation check, you plead with your physician to fill out the form, even if there is no real basis for the answers required. If the physician recognizes the subjective nature of the input, which they are providing, and prefers that it be done by qualified procedure, they become an obstacle to the system. The qualified facility where there are props to estimate weights lifted and simulation of job tasks that can be appropriately and objectively tested would consume overhead, employee time, and facilities; and, hence, a fee would necessarily be charged to the insurance carrier. Paying the fee would be quite appropriate if the information obtained is worthwhile; and, specifically, objective information should be well worth the cost. In any case, along with job counseling are testing for aptitude and other matters that may specifically benefit from a separate professional's input. Various states have several agencies that seek to retrain workers, provide assistance in various limited forms, and although budgetary crises and overall poor economic conditions diminish effectiveness, they may provide some valuable service, which may be of significant assistance to many workers, particularly those who may have been working at manual labor but have the aptitude and interest to be retrained or educated into other versatile careers that may be even more productive in our increasingly complex and technological society. While manual laboring may not be an option for some of these patients, less and less manual laboring is demanded in our workforce.

An occupational therapist may be essential in the evaluation of functional capacities since this is an occupational matter and involves testing and training to reachieve maximum function. A physical therapist may be necessary to provide back school, posture, and mechanisms of lifting, exercises, and work hardening. To understand more clearly the need for this comprehensive program and a menu which includes this form of treatment beyond the customary physical therapy, medication, exercises, and even surgical treatment, we need to consider next the concept of chronic pain.

PAIN PROGRAM

Patients who have chronic pain require specific intervention such as a pain program. When we consider the uncluttered and straightforward treatments for the physical problem of back injury, we will emphasize in the next chapter the fact that chronic pain may be present without any of these physical residual signs of injury. As such, we not only have the stress economically of the compensation case dispute and the uncertainty involved for the employee with a system which was designed to ensure continuity of one's income, but without any hope as there are no raises on compensation and, also, the continued suffering which interferes with family and recreation as well as occupation. Considerable discussion in previous chapters has pointed out the fact that we are dealing with a disability, the inability to return to work or enjoy one's lifestyle, recreation, and family; and this, specifically, is influenced by expectations, not only of performance but also of advancement and status among fellow workers and stresses, both on the job as well as within the person's personal affairs. Recognizing that we are not able to cure everyone, physicions have to be realistic at the beginning and not take it personally that a patient fails to improve despite good treatment. Rather than reacting against that patient as being a bad patient or uncooperative, we need to recognize that they may require the treatment of a team of professionals who have multidisciplinary resources and talents to provide. Accommodation by light duty or vocational retraining may be the most appropriate treatment, particularly for a patient who has chronic pain, as we will discuss in the following chapter. Chronic pain may prevent return to work and result in work hardening being ineffective in improving functional capacities for that patient to lift the number of pounds that is required for their particular job; and, thus, we need a comprehensive program that will deal with the problems that do arise. In this setting, a pain program is essential to deliver the comprehensive services required as opposed to hospice or other appropriate programs for terminal illnesses or other humane forms of treatment for chronic pain. If all physical treatments have been rendered and pain remains, treatment of the pain must be the subsequent focus, and this is the motivation behind pain clinics. Unfortunately, patients referred to the pain clinic would prefer to tell their friends that they have a herniated disc rather than chronic pain syndrome, so this author is of the opinion that an integrated program for pain management and functional restoration is most effective.

Included in such a program are psychological services which are intimidating to the patient who feels that the recommendation for such treatment is an accusation that the pain is all in their head. Further, psychological services or psychological support may be interpreted by the insurance carrier as an underlying complication that is the patient's fault and which mitigates their liability for the disability claim. On the other hand, disability and disappointment with regard to advancement, promotion, and loss of expectations can be depressing, may require refocusing on the future and the prospect of enjoyment for the remainder of one's career and life, rather than getting even for an injury sustained or treatment withheld, as many worker's compensation patients develop hostility and rage about how they are treated by the employer that they had faithfully been with for many years. The stresses of being unable to work causes depression and psychological reactions that are normal responses to the situation and which may require significant psychological treatment. To deny resources for this aspect of the problem may induce failure despite other satisfactory treatment. As such, it is important to have an integrated program so that all of the essential services, to the extent necessary, can be provided.

Often behavioral pain management as part of a functional restoration program can induce the patient to succeed in increasing repetitions or weight lifting or other limits so that they are focusing on the goal of what they are doing and not focusing on the earlier goal of just relieving the pain or allowing pain to interfere with her continued success. Such programs have shown themselves effective in patients otherwise unrehabilitatable and historically chronically disabled. Programs in which physical therapy and work hardening or other customary treatments are provided without the integrated focus of a complete program will fail and sometimes condemn the patient to continued disability because of the recommendation that they failed a program of functional restoration, where it may have been the program that was inadequate. The psychological component may not only induce greater success rates but may have far lower recurrence rates for subsequent disability and continued medical costs. Perhaps the reluctance of the insurance industry to cover the psychological component has some basis in the fact that it may be a Pandora's box that could lead to an endless string of bills for psychological treatment, but I think this is adequately addressed by making the psychological support part of a complete menu for a functional restoration or rehabilitation program, as shown in the literature and as necessary for patients with chronic disability and chronic pain. While the first time we swing a bat in the summer or weed the garden we have a tendency to get a blister, we do not give up on those activities; and, in fact, we develop a callous before the summer is over and are able not only to spend long times playing softball at church picnics but also to do all the gardening that is necessary; and, perhaps, this might give us an idea of what functional restoration really is all about. From this example, we can see the pitfalls in which the pain that results from doing certain exercises may lead the doctor or the therapist to say, "Stop those," whereas we really should continue. The following chapter will explain the concept of chronic pain that is in large part the reason a functional restoration program is necessary and needs to be comprehensive and completely outfitted in all its component parts.

Chapter 6

PAIN

Chronic pain is a very real experience of discomfort which is separated from acute pain by the predominance of an accompanying behavioral disorder where the pain comes to dominate the life of the patient who is preoccupied by a widening array of symptoms which may actually worsen with effective conventional treatment.

As we consider pain in the back, in medical parlance, we are dealing with a symptom. That is, the patient complains of a subjective experience of having pain. This report of pain then leads the physician to analyze the situation and apply certain examination techniques and tests to arrive at a diagnosis. Based upon that diagnosis, treatment should rationally follow to correct the underlying problem that is causing pain. We already have mentioned the fact that there is not in every case an identifiable pathoanatomic (pathologic or sick, and that of a specific anatomic location) source of the pain; that is, there is not a lesion we can point to and say it is the problem, as we would in appendicitis say that the appendix is what's causing the problem. Remove the appendix and the pain will be eliminated.

Our concept of pain has to be evaluated from an overall standpoint, not only to differentiate acute from chronic pain (and that will be the main thrust of this chapter), but we need to recognize certain fallacies in the thinking process. The first is that we usually expect that we can in a stepwise manner without overlap wait for the pain to go away and then subsequently, as achieving another rung on a ladder or step in a staircase, start rehabilitation. This may seem true or at least seem feasible for many injuries; however, it is not actually true in most cases. For example, if you have an ankle sprain, most people start walking before it is totally pain free. When a person is relatively comfortable and the pain is tolerable, and confidence has been gained through improvement up to that point (it is not going to take a bad turn and get worse), a person is then encouraged to go ahead and start walking on it. The confidence that it will continue to improve and that the pain will lessen in time allows resumption of function and as we use the leg or ankle, it gradually is rehabilitated by normal use back to a pain-free normal situation. Although we may have some trepidation and we would not proceed if warned by our doctor to wait longer, we feel that we are better rather than cured and at this point we start to resume normal activities.

There is a point at which most patients seem to arrive at the conclusion that they need to seek medical attention, and that is when they are not confident that things will continue to improve so that they can gradually resume their normal activities. There remains some trepidation and as they present to the doctor in cases in which it didn't work out, they will often say they thought it was all right, but they elected to proceed to have it checked out.

Unfortunately, the doctor cannot quantitatively gauge what "better" means and this is particularly the case many times when the patient is under treatment. Either the physician or, perhaps, the physical therapist may advise the patient to discontinue all treatment such as physical therapy because they still have pain, and encourage them to wait out the pain until it is completely gone, and then resume activities only after the pain is completely eliminated. This is because the definition of "better" is rather indistinct and being better does not mean that you have no further pain. Unfortunately, it seems that problems with the back carry a connotation of being under a black cloud and some people are reluctant to resume lifting or any relatively normal activities while they are still feeling the least amount of pain or simply stiffness after an injury, even if it may be remarkably less than it had been previously. This is also the case in many situations when the patient is actually in treatment. Unfortunately, the doctor is in a poor position to gauge improvement, other than by the patient's statements or reports of pain; and, in fact, they have to be recognized as being subjective, not objectively measured or tested, but simply what the patient tells the doctor. Often, when the patient calls the doctor and complains that they feel worse, the doctor will immediately say to stop everything, or the physical therapist, when hearing the report of worsening pain, will discontinue treatment until the patient sees the doctor again.

Waiting out the pain and then spontaneously starting activities only after the pain is completely gone is the situation that seems reserved for the back or for cases under treatment. Although we will discuss chronic pain in detail later, we have to recognize that chronic pain does not have objective findings in most cases and that the pain may never totally resolve. The patient's anxiety about returning to work and having the pain possibly worsen, as it may have on previous attempts, adds to the stress which may be present by conflicts between the employer and the employee, certainly not improved by a period of disability. It is then absolutely impossible to get the patient back to a point where they are not only totally pain free but are assured with a guarantee that they will not only have no pain or tolerable pain, nor that they will succeed if they return to their regular job. We don't require a guarantee that we will never again have a common cold as we are recovering from the cold and we return to work with the comment that we are better and should be fine in a few days. In fact, many people have frequent recurrent common colds and are told that they should stop smoking, but they not only suffer through the common colds and fail to improve in a few days as people otherwise normally do, but they not only live with it, they live with a chronic recurring partial disability and the potential for serious heart and lung disease as a consequence of their smoking. The smoking is voluntary but injury to the spine on the job is not something that we elected to have happen to us, so people are not psychologically prepared to accept the disability or the potential for recurrence for the case of a problem that has been imposed upon them.

This situation is further complicated by the difficulty that is part of the diagnostic process. When a patient has a fever, we seek to diagnose the source. We get a culture to see whether the sore throat is a result of having a strep infection that will benefit by treatment with penicillin or other antibiotics. While Tylenol may reduce the fever and relieve some of the symptoms, the streptococcal organism will remain unless antibiotics are used and has the potential for serious late sequelae and complications, such as rheumatic fever, unless penicillin is prescribed. It is widely understood that people should have rheumatic fever because of the widespread early use of penicillin and the appropriate seeking of a specific diagnosis, particularly through a throat culture. To complete the analogy with back problems, while a tonsillectomy may be recommended for recurrent strep throats as an assist to prevent these problems, it is not recommended for recurrent viral upper respiratory infection, even if severe.

With low back pain, the absence of a disc herniation on imaging studies represents the absence of an indication to consider surgery; however, the patient complains bitterly and persistently to the surgeon who then feels compelled to proceed with exploratory surgery (never helpful!) with the erroneous justification that perhaps it will help and that, if not, someone else will do it. They can only be disappointed when they find that a small disc herniation is not causing a large problem. As we have discussed earlier, the small herniation is not predicted to have benefit for any patient who seeks an operation without adequate indications. Perhaps this partly returns to the issue of fault; that is, if a patient has had an injury as a result of someone else's negligence, oil on the floor, or failing to obey safety rules, it is difficult for the injured person who is in pain and unable not only to work but to enjoy her normal recreation, her family, and lifestyle, to understand why she shouldn't be compensated, to be restored to a normal situation she had enjoyed previously. The analogy remains of the rusty fender: when the car is struck by another motorist, we feel entitled not only to a new fender but perhaps a rental car in the meantime whereas if the rust or "natural causes" (aging and arthritis) are responsible, then we understand that we need to accept the situation or get another car.

Low back pain does not have a similar pathoanatomic basis that we can definitively discover in each patient. As a consequence, physicians may find it convenient to describe the problem in terms of their bias or prejudice. While some physicians may ascribe the pain to a blown out disc, others may call it muscles and still others may call it ligaments and/or inflammation. It is indeed troubling for the patient who deals with these pseudoanatomic, illustrative not literal, causes for the pain and finds one doctor to give a different explanation from another. Because one doctor may say it's a disc and another may say it's a muscle, the patient feels confused and may even feel betrayed. This may lead to the patient feeling that he is not being dealt with above board, that he is being put off or not believed for the severity of the problem. Certainly the practice of medicine has suffered in recent years, and time spent with patients has been sacrificed for economies and balancing the federal budget. The reality is that these patients with back pain and anxiety take the most time for the least gratitude. If patients are already mad at their employer and mad at the bill collectors, then progressively get mad at their families, their friends, and the doctor, then even if you spend a lot of time they feel as if the doctor has not been willing to explain. When the explanations by some doctors differ from those by another, it is hard to convince the patient that the explanation really is too long for them realistically to understand and they would have to read the book, but that is the conclusion that I have accepted.

The medical model for pain is basically of a stimulus that is somewhere in the tissue and provides a signal to the brain, which is subsequently felt as pain. This is also called the acute pain model in which patients may, for example, have swelling of their thumb, having struck it with a hammer. Complete relief will be rendered from an anesthetic as the pain signals are interrupted, and although numbness is felt, pain will no longer be perceived. With appropriate time, healing, and sometimes treatment, problems that involve the acute pain model in some swollen or damaged area will recover and function essentially normally. In some cases it may be necessary from our medical model to diagnose and identify the pathoanatomic basis for the problem and thus direct the treatment specifically toward that problem. This is where we encounter a problem with chronic pain, since there commonly is not an acute pain source. What we are dealing with is called the chronic pain model. The problem then is what are we going to do when the pain does not go away either by itself or after treatment? With chronic pain we cannot wait out the experience of pain and then start the subsequent rehabilitation cycle. If we wait for the pain to go away completely, we will never get started in rehabilitation; and, in fact, the chronic pain problem is a cycle in which the actual swelling or tissue injury that caused the problem initially is no longer significant, but the perpetuation of the experience of pain is a very real, disabling, and vicious cycle. As a consequence, we need to analyze the situation that the patient involuntarily finds himself in and seek to minimize the pain by maximizing his function and distracting his focus from the pain to his potential to resume activities.

The problem we have then is, what are we going to do with the cases in which the pain doesn't go away? That is, if we have chronic pain, which is different from acute pain, we cannot wait out the pain and start the subsequent rehabilitation. If we wait for the pain to go away we will never get anywhere. Chronic pain is a cycle in which the actual cause of the pain is no longer significant, but the perpetuation of the pain is as a vicious circle that leads to disability. As a consequence, we need to analyze the situation that the patient finds herself in, and seek to optimize her function rather than focus on the pain.

Unfortunately, many patients with low back pain, and particularly those on disability, may not have an acute pain source, but fall into this chronic pain model. Minimal findings are present despite severe pain. This is specifically the reason we have emphasized that the severity of pain, whether acute or chronic, is not an indication to consider surgery. Unfortunately, treatment is generally based upon the patient's complaints that are an experience; and as the patient has suffering that is actually a behavior as a result of the pain experienced, rather than based upon the pathoanatomic lesion which is the basis for the pain, then the continued escalation of treatment to try to relieve the complaints would logically suggest surgical intervention. As surgery without proper indications is not aimed appropriately at a specific pathoanatomic lesion that can be cured, it is destined to be unhelpful. Hence, it is necessary to embark upon pain treatment that deals with the reality of chronic pain that can be severe and persist in the absence of a surgically removable lesion.

In this case, psychological approaches may be necessary, which is not to say that the problem is all in the head but, rather, that the problem is more a matter of coping than surgical. It is beneficial if the patient can then deal with the problem, and psychological techniques may be the most reasonable basis to provide relief and certainly are at least helpful in conjunction with other therapies. As such, we understand the lack of benefit of anti-inflammatory medications, as inflammation may have diminished and no longer be a principle component of the treatment. We, unfortunately, may find a great deal of iatrogenic, that is, physician-caused problems, where every time the patient has complained, the doctor has said to lie in bed or cease all function and activity. This is likely to result in contracture from inactivity and loss of muscle strength to the extent that pain is actually a result of such a perpetuated treatment that after a few days becomes inappropriate. Further, we see the lack of success in physical therapy and exercise, particularly when the patient is not actively participating as we have previously discussed, as the acute pain model is not acting; and,thus, there is no lesion to be relieved by exercise. Hence, the pain is perpetuated; and unless it is recognized as chronic pain and appropriate intervention instituted, the pain will continue unabated. Psychological support, unfortunately, may not be available as the insurance carrier would in many cases deny coverage; and although this probably has some merit as a Pandora's box of unlimited bills for psychological treatment may be opened, but failure to include psychological support as part of a pain program may predictably lead to failure for patients with chronic pain. This, in fact, is the experience of patients who have physical therapy, medication, and, unfortunately, even surgery; they are not better and they are chronically, completely, and totally disabled.

Many physicians may refer to this problem of chronic pain as having produced scar tissue in the area of concern. Although there may not have been an operation and there may not be what we customarily consider scar tissue, there certainly is a focus of some irritation that is then perpetuated, either by treatment or external stimuli. Acute pain seems to warn or protect individuals from harm or returning to activities that may cause further injury prematurely. Chronic pain from the same standpoint seems purposeless, as it does not show impending danger from a biological tissue damage standpoint, nor is it really protective except to prevent resumption of activities that may have caused the problem initially. Many cases are interpreted as emotional or social coping mechanisms as we would certainly want to be kind or at least sympathetic to an individual in pain. Particularly we would want to see them compensated for their needs in that they were unable to provide for themselves; and, particularly, as insurance companies seem large with resources that would not be strained for this suffering poor individual. If, however, they have chronic pain, this becomes exceedingly expensive, not because of the amount of the payment but because of the length. Many patients who are in pain, and the family has forgotten how severe the complaints have been, may find it necessary to go to the emergency room for some relief. Following this visit and the socially mandatory attention and accommodations, the patient finds some relief, even though from an objective medical standpoint the emergency room's contribution, other than status or declaration of the severity of the problem, is minimal. In other cases, the use of drugs will perpetuate a passive attitude and perhaps exacerbate depression, as most narcotics are mood altering and thus contribute to the problems of chronic pain.

The treatment for a chronic illness (which may include acute pain from arthritis, even if chronic) is seldom cure, but generally adaptations. We understand that arthritis can be successfully treated, for example, in a weight-bearing joint such as the hip, with a total joint replacement. That does not mean that we proceed at the first pain or with minimal limitation to a major replacement surgery. When the symptoms justify, replacement surgery is indicated, but certain limitations accompany that surgery. It is artificial and does not have the restorative potential of the God-given alive joint that was replaced because of damage. Similarly, patients who have had an operation should not be considered to be nineteen years old again, and may well have to accept permanent limitations as a result of the surgery. It is, nonetheless in some cases indicated that the surgery will relieve pain and be helpful, even if it will not return the patient to work. In perspective, it would seem reasonable then to provide adaptation or accommodations for an injured body part, when surgical correction will relieve some pain and restore some function, but will not make it entirely whole. For example, if a patient has a knee problem and is no longer able to drive a truck or bus with a hard clutch, we can either get a different vehicle or a different job and continue with that injured knee on a limited basis, or eventually operate and replace the knee and be unable to recommend, for care of the joint replacement, return to that job. Although return to that job is not possible, pain relief is gratifying. The same may occur in the spine where pain relief is obtained. However, return to heavy lifting and other activities is precluded by the damage that has already occurred, and the impairment which is permanent. It is a result of the impairment that the patient is disabled from certain activities, but the surgery is not for the disability. It is to benefit the impairment.

The problem of chronic pain is not a matter of relieving the pain. This is unlikely to occur and a poor prognosis can be predicted in advance if our focus remains on the pain rather than function. The reality is that the patient is not coping with the pain or with other circumstance as well, and this becomes the real need, namely, to cope with the pain, whether or not it is relieved. This is the basis of functional restoration that has been presented as a program or technique that can result in patients being able to perform physical tasks that they were previously unable to perform because of pain. What was noted within this program was that as the severity of the physical tasks are progressed in a carefully graduated manner, the pain increased only minimally and certainly not in proportion to the increase in physical demands. That is, doubling of the physical demand did not result in a doubling of the pain. On this basis, the patient was able to perform certain physical tasks despite the pain and as he progressively worked to perform more weight lifting or more repetitions in a task, he not only had the same pain but eventually was able to resume normal activities with less pain or having accepted the pain that was present so that it became less the focus of his attention. This was possible with significant psychological support as part of the program.

Patients may elect not to accept minimal pain, since they feel that it is abnormal and they were previously normal. Thus, they have decided that if they have any pain at all, they will not return to work because they previously did not have pain while they were working. Unfortunately, these patients are difficult to please and are truly unhappy persons. Patients who deal with pain and progressively increase their physical activities cannot only anticipate eventual restoration of satisfactory if not full function, but actual diminution in the severity of pain as all of their bodily systems, particularly the muscles and joints, resume function. Hence, the discs and joints resume nutrition through motion and the muscles reinforce the flow of blood and the exuding of metabolic waste products by an increased blood flow through activity and exercise. While this includes a psychological unfocusing or distraction from the physical problem, it is nonetheless only possible through a comprehensive team approach that attempts to restore function in disabled workers.

We also have to be aware that low back pain resulting in disability represents an entirely different problem. A headache may be an inconvenience on the way to a baseball game, but completely disabling for Saturday's lawn or garden chores or spring cleaning. Patients who are depressed may have pain in their back simply from the position that they are prone to assume when in a depressed mood, and patients who have marked stress on their job may find postural back pain unbearable. In fact, a majority of patients who are depressed will have pain in their back. As we consider the fact that back pain and disability are an evident and understandable cause of depression, recovery then becomes as much a matter of increased self-esteem that would relieve depression from increased activities as it is a matter of increased blood flow and relaxation of tight muscles after exercise that would relieve pain from lack of function.

In a case where there is severe job stress, an operation to remove disc material anatomically will not affect the stress on the job; and we may find a patient whose surgical technique was impeccable, whose nerve root pressure was completely eliminated, but whose disability was unaffected. It is self-evident that these patients are not aware of the true problem and, unfortunately, physicians are often unaware as well. The physician is frustrated to try to explain the bad result and the patient is willing to accept her surgery as having a bad result, even though technically it was flawless. The physician cannot explain the lack of benefit; and it remains a matter of denial on the part of the patient, who is really under stress, that it is the major problem. In fact, the physician who asks, "What's it like on your job?" is likely to get either a scathing response from the patient, or "Don't you understand how bad my back pain is?" Patients are often defensive in this regard and cling to the anatomic problem of a bad disc or some other problem, since that is the common ground they have with the surgeon, namely, that the surgeon's diagnosis is of an anatomic lesion for surgical cure. This may make it difficult for the patient to accept the need for psychological support or a pain program as the chronic pain diagnosis is not as impressive to their friends as having a blown out disc. Hence, the surgeon sometimes is the preferred caretaker of patients even when they don't have a surgical need.

This flattery is hard for some physicians to resist. Surgeons, of course, have personalities like other professionals. It is to be recognized that a boundless ego is not unusual in a surgeon; and as people they may be confident, self-assured, and easy to get along with, such that there may be a rapport with particular patients as their personalities intertwine. One problem that occasionally seems to be present is that some surgeons fail to have the self-confidence that patients anticipate and rely upon, as they place their trust in that individual to operate on their bodies. A surgeon who is not confident has difficulty engendering trust and, in fact, patients may have more complications. I have personally felt that confidence is a result of good training and being aware that technically you are as well able to perform any particular procedure as another surgeon, and so the services you are offering from a technical standpoint are on a par with those offered anywhere. Hence, you can tell the patient that you will do that surgical procedure and any complications that may occur are unavoidable. Some surgeons seem to find problems within their patients (problem patients) which are the cause of all the complications they encounter, whether they are technically up to date or able with confidence to say honestly that they are doing the proposed procedure as well as it is offered in any other setting. This is true, of course, for nonsurgical patients. Medical doctors who have read the current literature and know the range of diagnoses available and the tests necessary to determine the diagnosis that will guide subsequent treatment should be confident in their knowledge, training, and facilities. The attitude that is certainly a part of the underlying personality of some physicians— that they have bad patients and that bad patients have bad results— is certainly seen from time to time. Some of these individuals perhaps would have been happier in a profession other than surgery even if their parents (particularly some surgeon parents) strongly are pressing toward this noble goal of being a surgeon. We have to understand, however, that the patient may have problems, but the doctor's role is to help with those problems from the resources of his training of the medical profession's knowledge and research and scientific base and offer up-to-date care, not blaming the patient for bad results. Further, the physician needs to be in a position in which he can react as a professional to the patient whose suffering causes hostility toward many persons, including her doctor.

As physicians we feel that we are in many cases the last resort for many of these patients. Chronic pain seems to be self-perpetuating and in itself is addictive. The physician is the one who becomes the rescuer of these troubled persons. When they have a problem, they go to the doctor, get some medication, and then they subsequently restrict their activities and deal with the problem. As such, we need to reconsider the passivity role and failure to cope, but most of all, recognize that pain on a chronic basis is depressing, is stressful, and demands a comprehensive program approach.

While we see good results published as a result of functional restoration programs, and this may be a confirmation that some patients will benefit from psychological support or even psychiatric help, we recognize that this is not an underlying primarily psychological problem. That is, the patient did not necessarily have a psychological problem prior to the injury, prior to his present and future being threatened by his inability to work and to maintain his expectations, his future income, and provision for his family, and the fear and intimidation of being unable to continue on the job. Certainly psychological support would be appropriate for this situational stress and, perhaps, situational depression is inevitable as a result of chronic pain. In this perspective, we understand the quote from 1926 that "exaggeration of symptoms is as common as malingering is rare." Fellow workers have the impression that a person off with a back injury is not interested in working, but in an easy way out. Patients who have back pain understand that it is not easy to forego all of your plans, ambitions, and joys from working, being part of the crew, and having a steady reliable income, but the invisibility of back pain and, indeed, the absence of an acute pain model pathoanatomic lesion leads to these sorts of conclusions.

Certainly any person who had a motor vehicle accident before no-fault insurance, when it took six years to settle a case, understands the motivation not only for the no-fault laws that were to prevent the irreparable scars from the disruption that occurred after the accident. But if this would be your income rather than transportation, the inadequacy of the legal system to provide a timely solution based upon a law that was intended to continue an injured worker's income without disruption becomes evident. Certainly it does not take any cynicism or imagination to understand how legal manipulation can put the injured worker into severe economic distress as a means to try to force a settlement advantage. While the system deals this way, compensation patients may find it unfair and unreasonable that their assured benefits are interrupted because of contentions by the insurance carrier, which seem to the employee unfounded. While they feel and know that they have pain, they are being videotaped while walking to the store! They find themselves being questioned, as if committing a crime, and then being doubted and accused in a court of law of gaining through deception what they consider a fairly paltry sum from their former friend and loyal employer. The perspective we need to maintain is that the problem is actually that this disability causes more suffering than the back pain and, hence, our treatment needs to be directed toward that problem. When we deal with a disability, we understand the need for a multidisciplinary complicated approach rather than the surgical or medical cure for inflammation or a disc rupture or a spur. Where these anatomic problems can be solved easily compared to the interrelated complicated problems of disability, a complicated treatment program is necessary with the various expertise of multiple physicians trying to solve the true problem rather than the stated problem of low back pain.

Another confirmation of the fact that this is a problem involving components other than just the physical problem of pain in the back is the results of behavioral modification of pain. For example, it has been shown that when the first level manager or immediate supervisor of an employee calls and shows concern, this has been effective in minimizing lost time at various large companies, where it has been employed, to the extent of at least fifty percent reduction in cost for lost time in work injuries. This shows that the patient is worth having back and that he is missed by his fellow workers and, certainly with this attitude, he would be more assured of being able to return to work as a person recovering from the common cold might return prior to complete restoration but able to do their job, or at least ease into the routine gradually. On the other hand, I have often encountered the busy first line manager who insists that the employee does not return until they are restored to 100 percent. In this case, which is frequent in my experience , the boss does not want to be bothered by any accommodations for this injured worker. They have already been troubled enough by the absence and now they want the patient fixed by the doctor so that she can get on with her job. Understanding the fact that not all workers are still twenty-one years old, and that not all spines will be restorable, as many other body parts do deteriorate, we need to understand that some individuals require adaptation for chronic pain and will not be cured. In these cases, adamancy on the part of the immediate supervisor to be 100 percent before returning is almost a guarantee that the patient will be unable to return to the stress of that situation. Namely, do your job or get out. No worker is eager to return when he feels that the back pain may interfere with his productivity and performance on the job and, thus, being unable to satisfy the boss, risk termination and disgrace rather than continued compensation on disability. Certainly, if the patient could go to sleep and wake up after surgery cured, this would be ideal and certainly would be in the best scenario for the employer who wants the employee back productive as if nothing ever happened. This routinely happens; but, unfortunately, we become aware after investigation that eighty-five percent of the costs of worker's compensation are generated by fifteen percent of the workers: and as such, it is the few who do not fit this model who are intimidated at the thought of returning and then being unable to perform satisfactorily, who need to have psychological or job function support so that they can return assured that they will continue to have a job.

Finally, we see a lot of physical therapy facilities being opened as entrepreneurial ventures. These may have exercise machines and be called work hardening or fitness centers. As such, we see a lot of failures when psychological support is not an integral part of physical therapy. As a consequence, we see an acute modality used on chronic pain and can predict large numbers of failures. Thus, we would question the advisability of embarking on work hardening programs that are not comprehensive. We have seen in the literature the effectiveness of functional restoration and of a comprehensive program. When the program emulates mechanically a program in terms of a physical therapist and exercise machines, but does not have the facilities necessary to provide psychological support, vocational rehabilitation, and other matters, we cannot expect the same results as the complete programs reported in the literature. For this reason the referring physician has to be careful or, at least, aware that not every work hardening program can provide the resources required to work harden patients. Certainly, some patients will benefit from the exercises, return to work, and be grateful for the assistance. The problem that we have is that the chronic pain consumes enormous resources and is most likely to fail from a partial program. The recognition and awareness of what chronic pain constitutes should further illustrate the necessity of a complete program. The treating physician may have a personality that will or will not coincide with the desires and needs of that particular patient. Many physicians of great stature will not find certain patients to appreciate their style regardless of their capabilities. But beyond matters of style and personality, a patient will likely cling to the physician such as the surgeon who has an organic diagnosis and basis for her treatment, and when referred to other physicians, will decide sometimes on unrelated grounds whether that physician was helpful and whether or not they fully cooperate. The problem I have experienced is that a patient may be set for pain blocks or for psychological support and return with complaints about those providers who might have had significant extensive experience and who have been helpful with others. This does not shake my confidence in those physicians, but demonstrates to me that the patient's lack of benefit may be from other causes. After investigating and excluding a surgical lesion, I am left with a patient for whom the appropriate treatments have proven ineffective and sometimes seeing a patient frequently who is interested in getting the problem over with and feels that surgery is the only answer for their problem. Because of these cases, it seems increasingly clear to me that a program is required in which the patient is treated by all the physicians of various specialties within the program, and then the patient does not have his or her attention directed toward a physician caring for him, but recognizes that the program is designed to help the patient help himself. When the patient drops the passive attitude and grasps hold of the need to become actively involved, then that patient will not look upon one or another physician as being ineffective and return to the one of her preference, but she will recognize her own role and view each of the physicians as cooperating with each other for her benefit rather than specialists whose services she may or may not require.

Recognition of the separate entity of chronic pain has occurred in recent years, but we are only recently learning how we can deal with this problem. Unfortunately, many patients either select or are prescribed acute pain formulas. Patients who have had pain for many years, when they feel for whatever reason the pain has gotten worse, seek to have stronger analgesics or even stronger narcotics. As such, they are not dealing with the problem, but leaving it passively for the physician to treat. Further, a problem that is chronic by definition should not be treated with narcotics, which are by their nature addictive. As a consequence, the request for narcotics is inappropriate and contraindicated; but when the physician resists, the patient may become defensive about not abusing such drugs. The patient may become tearful as he feels he is not believed or he is not being compassionately cared for, and may even say to the physician, "Doctor, if you only knew how bad the pain was, you wouldn't say that I can't have those drugs." This, of course, is coupled with the patient who flatters the doctor about how good her care is and how the other physicians didn't understand how bad it was and hence the current doctor was the only one that recognized how severe the pain was and prescribed adequate medication— addictive narcotics for a chronic problem.

As a physician, I find it difficult to get insurance approval of referrals of patients to other specialists, even those whose services were clearly needed. This is particularly true as a surgeon. The diagnosis I supply is organic. It is an anatomic structure such as a disc that can be seen on X ray, which can be surgically manipulated, and which is psychologically unthreatening to the patient. If the patient is having difficulty coping with the problem and is referred for temporary benefit from injections, these results are still organic, but when the patient is relieved to the extent that he might return to work, the realization of what returning to work really means, perhaps unconsciously the job stress and other factors leads him to have objections to the anesthesiologist's treatment, rather than to the surgeon's analysis of the problem. More particularly, if he is referred for psychological support, the psychological problems are not something that we advertise to our friends, relatives, coworkers, and others who would find them a sign of character faults or other socially unacceptable views. As such, we don't want to be a wimp back on the job; and, so, when the psychologist is not supported by the insurance company, we are perhaps relieved because we are left with an organic problem preventing our return to work and are just unfortunate rather than unable to cope.

I hope that this chapter has helped explain that there is an entity referred to as chronic pain and although I have avoided a technical description or discussion of exactly what that may be, as it is beyond the scope of this book, I hope that the remarks that I have made will not seem critical of the patient or of the insurance carrier except to the extent that six blind men describing an elephant were all correct but all wrong as to what an elephant was really like. When we each see the problem from an isolated tunnel-vision perspective, we are going to contradict each other and the blind man holding the elephant's leg and describing the elephant as a tree as opposed to the man holding the trunk and describing the elephant like a rope may argue about the nature of an elephant. While both are correct, all they need to do to agree or to understand their differences is to open their eyes. Being blind they cannot. Hopefully, the readers of this book will have some increase in their vision from a humble physician who is trying to enlarge a practice of bringing together patient and insurance carrier while maintaining his own sanity and still seeking surgical patients for his practice. Next, we would like to discuss issues of posture and position as these are important: and we are getting away from strictly injuries of significant severity but rather overuse or chronic misuse of the body, which can cause pain.

Chapter 7

POSTURE

It's not a good position I am in. If I had to do the whole thing over again, I wouldn't.

—John Berryman

Attention to posture is clearly one of those treatments that many patients feel is a medicine that doesn't taste bad enough to be effective for them. As such, we have a lot of noncompliance with the recommendations for posture. Nonetheless, it is clearly a significant cause of pain in many persons, namely, that they may sit for long periods with their fingers on the home keys of a computer or typewriter and, as such, give little motion to the muscles between the shoulder blades (rhomboids) and have pain in that area. Stretching exercises can be effective, but seem inadequate to many patients for such a difficult problem. Patients who talk on the phone may have a neck ache and patients who do significant sitting, such as driving vehicles, executives at a desk, telephone operators, and others, can have a high incidence of low back pain from the posture involved in sitting, particularly if unsupported without an adequate lumbar support. Clearly, patients who are depressed will have poor posture; and, in fact, the majority of those patients will have low back pain as a result of depression. Most would like to have some medication to escape from their problems and, of course, desire those medications because of the pain in their low back. Patients who are unable to return to work will inevitably become depressed, and although not as dramatically as patients whose primary problem is that they are clinically depressed, this will be a component of not only the pain but also of a posture problem. Clearly, muscular exercise and recreational activities will increase our muscle tone and benefit our posture as well as our psychological condition and self-esteem; and, consequently, our mood will have considerable influence on our posture and whether we have pain in the low back.

Little has been said in recent years about posture. In the past, physical therapists had included attention to posture. I can say that my formal training as an orthopedic surgeon, including subsequent reading on the development in spine surgery, has not paid any attention to matters of posture. This is certainly not to suggest that my teachers were ever easy on me or left out things that were customarily part of curriculum, but that posture has been neglected in recent years. Posture means the position that we assume over long periods of time, and good posture would suggest that we are treating our bodies well and not causing undue distress. A balanced posture would mean the earlobe is over the acromion or the point of the shoulder, and the point of the shoulder, if we are standing, is aligned over the greater trochanter, or the bump on the side of our hip, and then this would be centered over our lateral malleolus or outside ankle bone. Figure 14 illustrates what would be considered good posture. As we consider posture, I can recall my mother telling me to put my shoulders back and my head up, and I thought at the time, she was trying to show off her son and impart to me a posture related more to self-esteem than to prevention of back pain. In most cases it is unrealistic to explain posture in generic terms to a diverse audience. For example, a violinist has to assume a posture that allows proper bowing and positioning of the instrument. Orchestras will by necessity find either someone within their ranks to teach good posture to musicians or otherwise to refer to physicians who are specifically sensitive to this problem. Sports medicine physicians who take care of dancers, as in a ballet company, or other performers, similarly will need to be well informed with the specific activities involved and become specialized consultants bringing to bear their medical knowledge upon a special technique and situation they have learned about on the job. The customary sports medicine activities such as watching football games and attending to the injured on the sidelines, or basketball games or other activities, seem self evident. However, workers may have significant occupational postural pain and, hence, the spine doctor has to become equally familiar with the positions of work at specific jobs. Although physical therapists may make a great deal sometimes be called on along with industrial nurses to evaluate a particular workplace for its ergonomics, the doctor is no longer just providing a treatment based upon principles of anatomy and disease, but must become actively involved in the special activity the injured worker was performing.

Clearly this should, and eventually must, become part of the treatment of patients at work. Rehabilitation companies are becoming increasingly aware of the need to visit the job site, analyze the activities, and make specific recommendations for that employer. The entire field of ergonomics, or proper body mechanics, has advanced greatly in recent years in our understanding and knowledge. It is, however, unfortunate that the information and knowledge has not been transmitted to many workplaces. As a consequence, a lot of preventable problems continue to occur. As a physician, it is evident that there are a lot of employers who could greatly benefit but fail to recognize the potential. One patient in particular had severe pain, problems with degenerative arthritis, was overweight, and had diabetes. I operated on this patient who was improved but still had diabetes, was still significantly overweight, and had continued pain. He eventually went back to work after removal of arthritic spurs that were pressing on nerves, resolution of swelling and relief of the leg pain, but he was certainly not restored to full normal function. I had explained in detail prior to the surgical procedure that that was not to be expected, particularly in light of his diabetes which would make his heart, his kidneys, his circulation, and so on less than normal. At work, a particular manipulation of the part that he was machining had required him to stand up, to bend over further than was comfortable, and look to the opposite side of the part while in the machine. The installation of a mirror was of negligible cost compared to the wages of this person who had been out of work for many months prior to his surgery. Nonetheless, the employer was forced, kicking and screaming, by the insurance carrier to install that mirror. This allowed the patient to sit in a posture that would not cause recurrent pain and disability while effectively continuing to perform the manipulation and production that the employer desired.

Certain modifications are clearly possible. For example, when working at a lathe or another machine, a stool to put the foot on or alternately to move the pelvis and relieve tension from chronic unchanged positions can

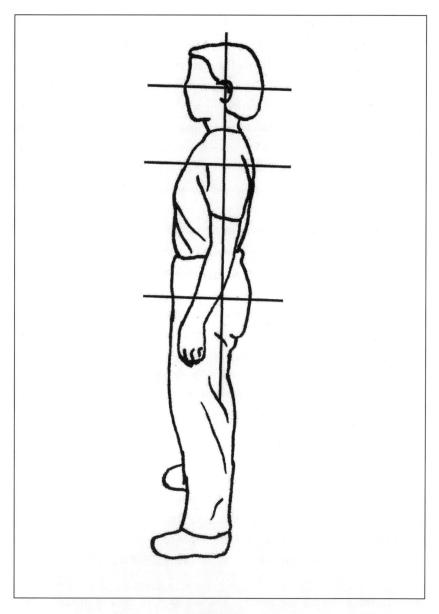

Figure 14

Good posture is demonstrated when the earlobe is over the acromion of the shoulder, which is then directly over the trochanter, relieving muscular tension on a postural, all day basis, by balance.

of difference. This certainly would be helpful for a patient behind the counter who could lean to one side and then the other and equally well fill out orders or handle customer needs. This is the reason bar rails are provided; but, of course, prolonged standing in that location can lead to other problems than just pain in the back.

The most important principle in terms of body mechanics really can be summarized partly with common sense. That principle is leverage. If the baby in the crib is to be lifted, then the baby should be brought to the near side of the crib and lifted close to the mother. If a worker has to reach a lever or pick up a part, accommodations should be made so that the repetitive function does not have to be done with the arms outstretched from the body. If parts have to be lifted out of a box which, for example, is three or four feet high so the worker has to reach over into the box, then the parts should all be brought near the wall of the box or, more reasonably, the sides of the box removed to prevent injury and stress on the back. We have discussed previously the muscular control needed to support the pelvis so that the lumbar spine will have a foundation on which to act. It seems clear in the same sense that if you lift up too much with a crane when the boom is down, you tip the crane over (Figure 15). To prevent tipping the crane over, you boom up. The back needs to have the boom raised; that is, the smaller the angle of forward inclination, the less the stresses are on the muscles in the lumbar spine and this requires no great calculation or computer analysis of forces in the low back. Further, it is clear from an understanding of the low back that the normal posture of lordosis is safe for the low back, so if a heavy weight is to be lifted, the knees should be bent slightly so that the lordosis or bowing in of the low back is maintained. One look at the side view of a weight lifter lifting a heavy weight will convince a person of the need to bow in the back, as certainly with the extent of weights lifted by competitive athletes in weight lifting. Any deviation would cause serious injury and all participants will be noted to have the back bowed in when they lift.

As an extension of posture are the techniques of lifting, such as demonstrated by back schools or physical therapy sessions (Figure 16). These figures illustrate the way in which lifting should be done as well as some postures or lifting techniques that should be avoided. The science of ergonomics is developing and becoming increasingly important, where a patient should use certain techniques for lifting to minimize stresses on the discs and other structures in the back, and can predictably be injured by certain postures during manipulation of parts or in techniques of lifting. With computer-generated analyses of forces, we can become more specific about work situations that need to be modified for safety as opposed to the more coarse application of epidemiologically discovered risk factors.

If we were to consider lifting in its most stressful case, we would look at weight lifters and the techniques they use. First, a weight lifter's belt is a lumbosacral support. In the same sense that flexion exercises sought to strengthen abdominal muscles, the weight lifter's belt supports the abdominal muscles, which are stressed during the peak of the lift.

Next we notice that the weight lifter will always maintain a modest lordosis in the spine while lifting, and we would expect this position (as opposed to a forward flexed position) to prevent undue stresses on the disc between the vertebral endplates as we have discussed before, as a ball bearing between two steel plates, as a matter of centralizing the load on the disc and not allowing an undue force propelling the disc toward the nerves in back. This position is important for all lifting; and, hence, we have the adage of bending the knees, which allows a position of the spine not only so that the muscles are not stretched out but the discs are in this neutral position. If we consider the muscles and ligaments of the back, they will not be understretched but will be relaxed in a lordotic position. Certainly a relaxed structure will be less vulnerable to injury such as overload, as it first has to be preloaded. If you want to tear a piece of paper, or a telephone book you first tense it, as you can't tear it in a relaxed position, and this analogy probably has some merit.

Translating this principle further, we have the problems of making a bed, in which the nature of the task requires bending over the bed and being at a mechanical disadvantage to perform this task. Clearly this is exacerbated by situations in which we cannot come around to the other side of the bed to make it or, optimally, have a second person pulling on the sheet on the other side, as in some cases is possible in the hospital setting. If we have a double bed and it is up against the wall, it is almost impossible to make that bed without getting on it; and we certainly will be in a disadvantaged position with the boom down while we try to position the

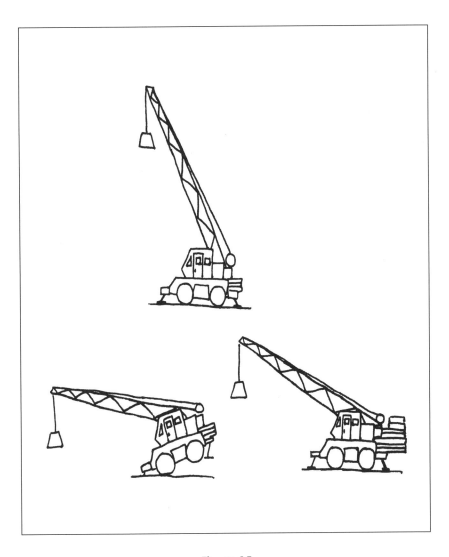

Figure 15

A crane illustrates lifting techniques. The boom up is a person who is more erect when lifting a heavy load. The boom down causes the crane to tip over, which means the load is not close to the body.

sheets appropriately. Clearly, many activities of daily living and around the home can be a particular problem unless we carefully consider body position in those activities. If we think in terms of the weight of a single sheet, this is not a heavy-duty task. However, if we look at the energy expended while making a bed, it is a significant physical exertion.

Another example might be lifting, which could be either suitcases for an airline, various parts on a manufacturing line, or delivered product that is unloaded from a truck. Each of these tasks requires some flexion of the lumbar spine and bending to pick up objects, but as the anatomic details of the lumbar spine reveal, the facet joints are oriented up and down so that rotation is not one of the intended or allowed movements. As such, twisting while lifting or picking tends to stress the facet joints significantly and probably contributes to the common facet syndrome or deterioration of the facets in the low back. Hence, picking up objects as Figure 16 illustrates and then pivoting with the object held rather than twisting the trunk would be highly recommended. Finally, pushing and pulling are analyzed in terms of position of the spine, whether in flexion or extension during the maneuver, and in Figure 17 and 18 we see recommended positions for pushing and pulling, with the intent of maintaining a normal lumbar lordosis. These positions particularly apply to the common problem of running a sweeper or vacuuming which, of course, is necessary in all households.

It is clear, however, that some postures are going to result in increased tension on the ligaments and muscles. Over the course of many hours, this increased tension will inevitably lead to pain from prolonged unchanged posture. This is in addition to the special problem of vibration that has been identified as a hazard to the spine for a salesman driving a car or a truck driver whose lifting and loading or unloading are independent problems in addition to the vibration of the road. Restricted motions that would occur from unchanged postures, most commonly the failure to be able to extend backward at the lumbosacral joint, will lead to increased tension on a constant postural basis from a contracture of soft tissues for patients who are commonly so involved. For these patients, the simple procedure of doing back bends, such as the program promoted by Robin MacKenzie, *Treat Your Own Back*, may result in an enormous improvement in back pain. However, less formally, just changing postures frequently should be of considerable assistance and good normal exercise.

Beyond the fact that pulling on something is inevitably going to result in pain from the increased or excessive tension, we must view the range of motion of the joints of the body as well as the spine as being options from which the brain can select a comfortable posture. This is a complicated integration of signals from all of the joints in terms of the proprioceptive nerves in each of the capsules and joint structures which is then put together for minimum tension overall and, hence, for comfort. Restrictions mean that the position of posture that the brain can select and supervise for the body loses options. Some of these options may be comfortable and some of the options remaining may be painful. Hence, we would suggest that it is simply logical that supple movable joints would lead to more comfort.

It has been interesting to me that in many cases when a patient is sitting on my examining table in the office, and I place one hand on a shoulder and press with the other hand on the small of the back to align the lumbar posture, the cervical posture automatically corrects itself. The consequence of the examiner gently guiding correct posture (normal lordosis) in the lumbar area shows the coupled nature of the overall balance of the spine. When one area changes, others respond so that we remain erect. It's as if we have a self-regulating or a self-balancing system in our spine. An appropriate position would align the ear over the acromion, or the point of the shoulder, and this alignment of the ear over the acromion would also be over the greater trochanter in the standing position. This posture allows balancing of the spine and minimal muscle activity to maintain that position.

As we discuss posture, we should also talk about sleeping. Many questions arise as to what is an appropriate or an inappropriate mattress. Further, a lot of people are concerned as to whether a waterbed, which often is presumed to be bad, would be totally unacceptable or a consideration. Some patients ask with significant timidity, which to me usually suggests that they already have a waterbed and they want to have some notion of how bad a thing they are doing to their back. The waterbed is not necessarily bad, and I find many surprised when I fail to condemn it.

The crux of the issue is actually the support of the spine. If we lie on a bed and the bed is too soft, we find that the support under the side does not

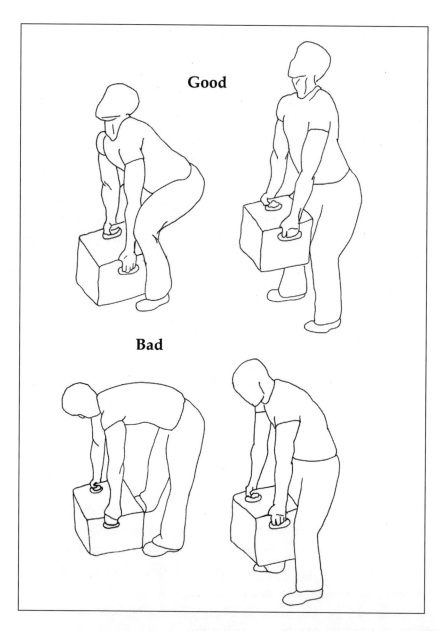

Good

Bad

Figure 16

Good lifting techniques involve having the back bowed in or a slight lordosis.
Bad lifting techniques have the back bowed out, or failure to maintain lordosis.
This causes undue stress on the back muscles.

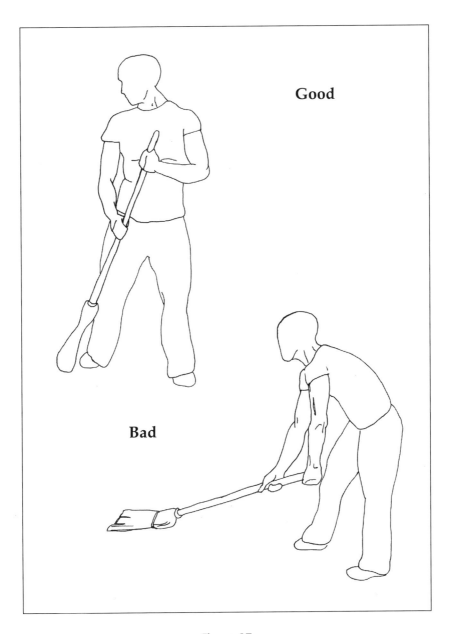

Figure 17

Activities such as sweeping, or any push and pull avtivities are illustrated as good techniques above with a lumbar lordosis, or poor techniques with failure to maintain lordosis.

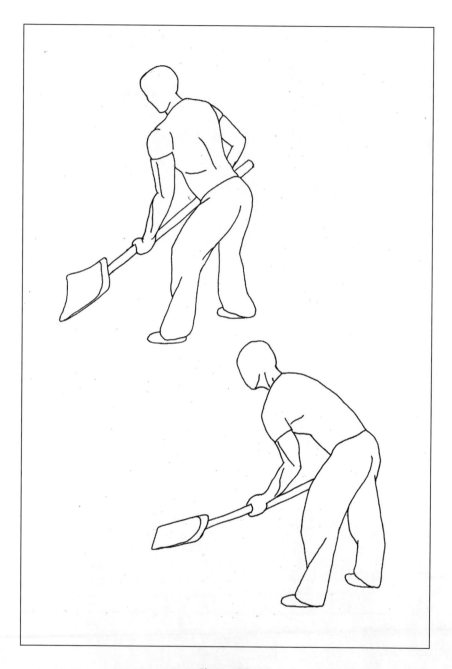

Figure 18

Shoveling with lordosis maintained is a good technique, whereas shoveling without the lordosis risks injuring the spine.

hold the spine up. If we were lying on our side, and someone took a line along the spinous processes or the middle of the back, we would see a curve of inadequate support or a bed too soft, as the hips and the shoulders sunk into the bed and the flank (or the side) was not supported, so that the spine sagged into a potentially painful position (Figure 19). Applying an indicator such as a strip of tape along the spine while standing straight would then demonstrate this principle of spine support; namely, if the spine is properly supported, the tape should be straight. If the bed is too soft then there will be sagging in the spine and we would expect the body weight to cause a backache in the morning from this constant stress on the spine throughout the night. If the bed were too hard, we would again see that the spine would sag and the shoulders and hip would not sink in, and again, the side of the body is not supported. If we were to place a pillow or, more feasibly just as a test, to roll up a towel and put it around our middle with a safety pin for sleeping at night to see if it should help, we then would have some support under the side, and this should allow adequate support, both lying on the side so that we can see our piece of tape as an indicator or when we lie on our back, which is somewhat more complicated to illustrate.

If we look at a water bed or a mattress with appropriate support (for which a water bed qualifies as a satisfactory example), we would then visualize someone lying on her side and the line drawn along the spinous processes or the bumps along her back while she is standing straight, would then be straight because of appropriate support for the spine while she is lying on her side of the bed. Hence beds can be too hard or too soft, and waterbeds may be fine. In the next chapter, we will discuss back pain as related to some positions in bed and, of concern for married persons experiencing back pain, how to obtain the normal enjoyment of sex while experiencing a backache. Also explained are consequences that the fruits of marriage produce—an increased lordosis and stress on the wife through the resulting pregnancy.

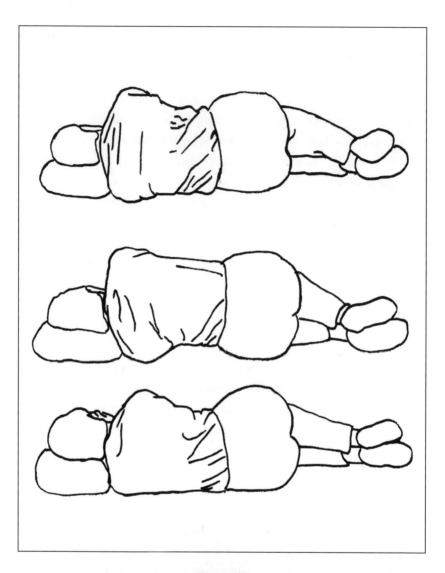

Figure 19

Top figure, spine is supported and in nuetral position. Middle figure, the surface is too soft and the pelvis and hips sink in, allowing a sag and strain on the spine. The bottom figure is for the surface being too hard and again, strain is placed on the low back.

Chapter 8

PREGNANCY

Lo, children are an heritage of the Lord and the fruit
of the womb is his reward.

—Psalm 127:3

When we consider the influence of backache on working people, we need to consider the incidence in the working population of pregnancy as a concomitant, increasingly prevalent disease, particularly as women become a more significant portion of the workforce in every aspect. Epidemiologic studies have suggested that a higher percentage of females who have had more pregnancies resulting in live births will have cases of acute herniated lumbar intervertebral discs than women who have had fewer pregnancies. That statistic would imply a risk associated with pregnancy of having a herniated disc. Unfortunately, the problem is not as simple as that may imply, since a herniated nucleus pulposus is actually rarely associated with pregnancy despite the fact that two-thirds of women have back pain with pregnancy and one-third continue to have pain even one year later. The usual and customary pain is actually in the sacroiliac joint. The hormone, relaxin, is released during pregnancy, preparing for a relaxation or laxity of the ligaments particularly in the symphasis pubis, that is, a connection of the pelvic bones in the front, which has to open to create the birth canal, as well as the sacroiliac joint. The sacroiliac joint has to bend open to allow the pelvis to open and thus to create the birth canal. As a consequence, low back pain occurs in the pregnant woman when the relaxin is in high concentration and ligaments get loose. That increase in concentration begins fairly early in pregnancy and, as a result, she experiences back pain. The relaxin diminishes quickly after delivery, but the back pain continues, because the sacroiliac joint and all the ligaments have to heal.

The increased incidence of herniated nucleus pulposus has been presumed to be the excess of stress of the pregnancy, or weight of the gravid uterus (filled with baby) but also includes the ligamentous laxity, again caused by the hormonal changes during and toward the end of pregnancy by the hormone, relaxin, which is from the corpus luteum and an added exacerbation beyond the mechanical stress of the fetus. Some women are afraid of becoming pregnant because of the fear of associated back pain or an injury to their back resulting from the pregnancy. Certainly other symptoms, such as carpal tunnel syndrome or venous problems in the legs, are highly associated with pregnancy and considered involved risks. Pregnancy has more commonly been treated by insurance in recent years as a disease. In the past, reimbursement of several hundred dollars as an award for pregnancy to cover the costs became so inadequate that even married couples planning for a child and setting aside money to pay the doctor and hospital found themselves with a bill they could not handle. As a consequence, most insurance companies were coerced into covering the pregnancy as an illness rather than this exclusion. Nonetheless, it is not a compensable injury or illness, although leave time is allowed and arrangements can be provided. Our need is, nonetheless, to learn not only how to continue productively during the condition of pregnancy, but also to return to work following delivery with the added stress of pregnancy's reward, the newborn.

Pregnant women often develop low back pain with pregnancy or have the exacerbation of prior and existing problems. Back pain is common with a majority of women, which may be in many cases a woman's first episode of low back pain since she is young and usually otherwise healthy. The risk of recurrence after delivery is elevated when back pain has been present during a previous pregnancy by as much as double the usual incidents. Presentation is commonly at the lumbosacral joint and particularly over the sacroiliac joint with some radiation into the buttocks. It may also be above the lumbar area toward the lumbosacral junction in some cases. The routine problem of pregnancy really is centered over the sacroiliac joint which is often, from lack of details, physical examination or history, lumped with disc herniation problems, as we have already discussed: the dynasty of the disc—everything is attributed to the disc, since it is the most common problem. Nonetheless, disc herniations may occur and there is an increased risk of disc herniation, which is associated with an increased number of previous pregnancies. However, the principle problem and the usual low back pain is in the sacroiliac joint which is stretched and relaxed by the maternal hormones and more mobile than customarily expected. The sacroiliac problem seems to be differentiated clinically from lumbosacral problems or disc problems because it specifically interferes with the ability to stand in place or to sit. Patients with disc problems have more difficulty with ambulation, particularly problems ascending stairs or walking up an incline.

The increase in lordosis which accompanies the weight of the fetus pulling the patient forward, subsequently requires the woman to lean backward to counterbalance that weight, as opposed to carrying the weight. It is much easier to balance it, but swayback or increased lordosis has been heavily associated with back problems and lumbar fatigue, including risk of disc herniations as well as strain of the muscles. Sacroiliac problems without pregnancy are often associated with a twisting type injury and there certainly are a lot of cases where a pregnant woman will have to twist or bend to get up because of awkwardness and the need to counterbalance the weight of the uterus and the fetus. There is fatigue and there are problems from twisting and bending that do not end, as the baby then has to be lifted and cared for, so these problems accumulate and lead to significant problems by the end of the pregnancy. Unfortunately, with the continued stress and the time interval it takes for the ligaments to heal, back pain from pregnancy does not always disappear as a result of delivery.

The natural history has been investigated in various populations and there are clearly several hypotheses, but also a number of factors, that enter. Clearly maternal age, the number of previous pregnancies, and hormonal levels have been shown in the literature to be important. In every case, an increase in the biomechanical load is seen on the spine with the forward bending movement of the weight of the fetus which has to be counterbalanced by increased extension or an increase in the lordosis of the woman during pregnancy. Lumbar tilt is clearly changed and the normal curve is distorted with the sacrum more horizontal. Shifting of this equilibrium requires the leaning back of the trunk and a partial straightening of the lumbar lordosis above, so the lordosis in the lower lumbar spine is not only increased but increased as a percentage of the total when it is a less symmetric distribution of curvature. The weight of the baby is associated with an increased stress in the spine; and this increased stress is particularly a problem because the collagenous tissues which support the structures are lax from relaxin, and this particularly affects the sacroiliac joint and the dense ligaments associated with pelvic stability. Medications are generally excluded because of their significant effects on the fetus. Corsets can be worn, but they have to allow room so they do not constrict circulation or otherwise cause swelling; and, particularly later in pregnancy, it is difficult to brace without causing excessive tension. The abdominal muscles and pelvic floor exercises are commonly employed and they are the most helpful; and they are then, after delivery, a necessity to resume normal, comfortable activities and function.

Sacroiliac problems either during pregnancy or postpartum are unlike low back pain, which is usually otherwise dominated by disc problems. Injuries to the pelvis involve disruption of a closed ring. That is, the two major pelvic bones are attached in front at the symphasis pubis and in back on each side of the sacrum by the sacroiliac joints and ligaments. The common injury to the pelvis is called an open book injury, where the sacrum is like the binding of a book and the iliac wings or the iliac bones are the pages and cover of the book. The symphasis is opened, as breaking a seal on a book that is being opened, such as a test booklet for an examination. If you break a pretzel, the pretzel has to crack in two areas since it is also a closed ring and, similarly, the pelvis basically has to have some soft tissue or bony injury in the front as well as in the back. The open book type pelvic injury can occur, for example, from passengers in an automobile thrown against an armrest or the door, opening the book.

From this model of the disruption of a closed ring such as the pelvis, it seems clear that if we wrap a belt around the pelvis, we will be closing the book. If the ligaments of the sacroiliac joint are loose, swollen, or partially torn, then compression circumferentially around the pelvis will put the matched ends of the joint surfaces in apposition (closer together) and relieve the stress on the healing ligaments. The sacroiliac belt is essentially such a treatment, in which a belt encircles the pelvis, usually over the trochanter, the bony bump on the side of the body where the muscles from the pelvis attach to the thigh bone or the femur. The belt can be placed either over the trochanter or above the trochanter, and below the rim or the crest of the ilium (the top of the pelvis which is basically your belt line). in that area (between the crest of the ilium and the trochanter) is a fleshy area of muscles, which can be compressed with a belt to "close the book" and relieve the pain on the sore healing ligaments from injury, trauma, or child-birth. The birth process represents an opening of the ring and if the pelvis opens in the front to provide room for the birth canal, clearly the sacroiliac joints have to move more than they normally move to allow the process of birthing. That opening is possible because of the gradual relaxation result-ing from the hormone, relaxin and from the force of the child's head during the labor phase. Basically, the ring is stretched open. Postpartum, the sym-phasis comes back together but ligaments heal over a period of time.

Laxity in the ligaments before delivery may be treated by a sacroiliac belt that would be around the hips and below the abdomen. This type of support should have less constrictive effect and, hence, less contribution to swelling in the legs whose venous outflow is already impeded by the weight of the uterus against the great vessels and veins in the pelvis, as it is outside of the bony structure and should not transmit pressure through the soft tissues as significantly as a properly placed low back brace or corset. Exercises performed postpartum are appropriate to restore the circulation, mobilize fluid, and strengthen muscles which in the pelvic area have been severely stretched and are clearly a more extensive process than just the healing of the surface of the uterus after the placenta comes off and the episeotomy. Customary low back exercises may be helpful to restore nor-mal spinal flexibility, muscle tone, and alignment after the distortion from the increased lower lumbar lordosis and upper lumbar lack of lordosis to counterbalance the weight of the fetus but general aerobic exercises are most helpful. Aerobic exercises are discussed elsewhere, but essentially increasing blood flow from muscular exercise with a slight increase in heart rate and working to the point of a light sweat maintained for fifteen or twenty minutes causes increased oxygen throughout the body. The resulting blood flow flushes out metabolites, relaxes stretched and sore muscles, and restore normal physiologic function through the increased circulation generally throughout the body.

Sacroiliac problems cause difficulty standing in place, since the weight of the spine, upper trunk, and body are transmitted through the sacrum to the pelvis through the sacroiliac joints. Standing in place is generally best interrupted by having a small stool or something to alternately put one leg on, then the other, while standing at the changing table, the sink, or at the kitchen counter so that the distribution of weight is shared and the change in position relieves the distress until it is time either to resume other activities or to find a rest position.

Prevention would be a desirable goal, and that is probably achieved by adapting lifestyle and, particularly, the work environment to reduce the loads on the spine. The exercise that may be the most important for the woman is to sit in a chair and bend forward to allow the accentuation of the lordosis to be decreased at least temporarily as she spreads her legs apart, to allow room for her to forward flex the spine in the upper part, which is a response to the fetus in the uterus. This change in position may be the most restful and provide considerable comfort. This is particularly important for women who have had previous back pain with their pregnancies and for whom a modification of heavy physical work can be accomplished. The second matter is one of education involving prophylactic back school to emphasize posture, working positions, lifting techniques, and methods to avoid or alleviate a backache. Finally, the third treatment would be to place the pregnant woman in a prophylactic corset or brace. These, however, cause enough problems so that it is difficult to recommend such a treatment for all women. Some may benefit; others experience a significant negative effect on the trunk muscles and the corset can be cumbersome. Problems with exacerbation of lower extremity swelling, in particular, may outweigh any potential benefits.

While pregnancy may interfere with sexual intercourse, it does not preclude it. As patients with back pain may have problems enjoying sex, they still can find some positions that will be possible to accomplish this goal. Certainly the rest positions and exercises that previously have been mentioned to relax the muscles in the back should be duplicated during sexual intercourse. The partner with back problems should, if possible, lie on her back with a pillow between the hips and lower back to provide lumbar lordosis and, if possible, the knees bent. This position is ideal for the woman for support of the back and relaxation of the muscles, but also lying on the side with hips and knees flexed with the husband in the same position behind can be satisfactory. Backache is second only to headache as a reason for not having sexual intercourse and certainly there is some stress on the muscles during sexual excitement and muscle tension, but this should not be extreme or exaggerated to the point of severe pain. Pain to the male with erection or ejaculation is not anticipated from the back and, hence, would be an indication to have the prostate and genitourinary organs examined by a urologist.

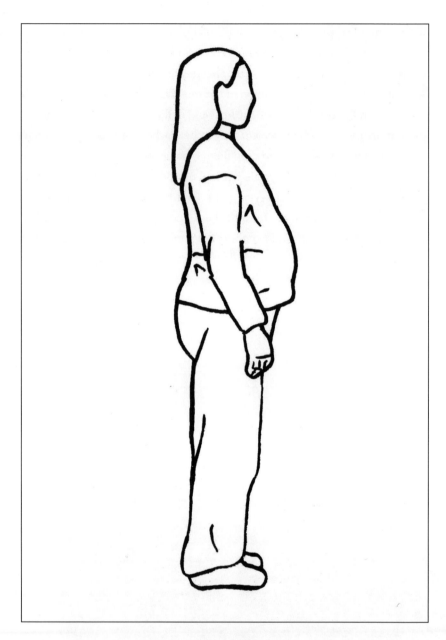

Figure 20

Pregnancy results in an increase in lordosis, or swayback, to position the head and trunk over the pelvis, and balance the gravid uterus.

Chapter 9

PREVENTION

A state is not a mere society, having a common place,
established for the prevention of mutual crime and for
the sake of exchange . . . political society exists for the sake of noble
actions, and not of mere companionship.

—Aristotle

The most important issue in any consideration of backache is how not to have it. Certainly an ounce of prevention is better than a pound of cure; and if we are serious about preventing back pain, we should review what is known. We have discussed the fact that an active involvement in physical fitness and aerobic health can prevent pain, minimize disability, and allow more rapid response to treatment and recovery. The real problem is not preventing backache from ever happening, as this may not be possible, but to prevent the disability that may accompany back pain and result in severe complications that we have discussed. This is particularly significant since the backache we may need to treat carries with it an expectation that it may recur in about forty percent of cases within the first two years. Specifically, we need to know what to do when there is a backache to get it behind us, to work with it, and to minimize its influence on our activities. We also have discussed the importance of posture for preventing increased tension through the course of a day on muscle groups, which will then be painful at the end of the day. We have also discussed the fact that pressures in the disc are higher in the sitting position than they are standing, and although this may not be helpful to people who drive, such as salesmen or truck drivers, a lumbar support can reduce this pressure and alternating positions can be helpful in preventing severe problems in the back.

Unless we are prevention oriented, we are likely to have problems that become severe before we take appropriate action and this can result in unnecessary interruption of our schedules. We are far more likely to change oil when the car computer tells us that it is due for an oil change than to remember to look at the odometer, and we are certainly far more likely to do exercises for good health when we start to have a problem. When glucose tolerance is impaired, we are forced to diet appropriately because the alternatives are far worse. When blood pressure starts to go up, we are convinced that restricting our salt intake is less troublesome than medication or the potential complications of those medications. When we have chronic cough and frequent colds, we will consider the suggestion of giving up smoking, but the lack of immediate reinforcement and usually denial on the part of the smoker along with the failure to recognize the extent to which this is a behavioral problem, causes difficulty in accomplishing that. When we have to buy the next size waist in our trousers, we consider going on a diet. Until our neck hurts from talking on the phone with the cradle against our shoulder, we neglect the good advice, that had been given to us in health class in school or perhaps by physicians or family or friends. Unless the importance of prevention is recognized even when we don't have a problem, we may suffer needlessly; therefore, this discussion is intended to reinforce our awareness of the need to seek to avoid problems.

If we consider the seated position (Figure 6), this is not different from the position standing and bending over at 90°, except that our knees are bent. The standing position in that much forward flexion looks painful, but what we don't recognize is that this is the same position with regard to the lumbosacral joint as sitting represents. As such, we should recognize the need while sitting to get up from time to time and do back bends or to allow our motion of the spine to be restored and to prevent chronic stress, which will be the cause of stiffness. Further, this will result in us arising from a seated position after a long interval in a forward flexed position. This is commonly seen as a consequence of driving long distances, because we are sitting for a long time. When we arise from the car, we will be in a forward flexed stiffened position. Changes in posture can be important under these particular circumstances, that is, the back bend exercises will provide a posture not achieved otherwise, and they prevent us from being contracted in that forward flexed position, such that the erect position (when we resume standing) is our position of maximum extension. If we can extend such that we bend backward 30%, then coming up from the seated or forward flexed position will not be a problem as the erect position is no longer the limit of our range of motion.

As we have discussed previously, nutrition to the disc only occurs during motion. When movement occurs and the influence of gravity or the stress of muscle action changes, water is either drawn in by the osmotic pressure of the proteoglycan molecules and exchanged with nutrients, or it is extruded by the stress of the muscles and gravity. These cycles of nutrition for the disc are essential and the only way that needed solutes can get into the disc space. Unfortunately, the metabolic activity, as we have mentioned, is interrupted by cigarette smoking, where the oxygen tension in the disc is cut in half within the disc just by lighting a cigarette, and can be maintained at that low level by having merely three cigarettes over the course of a single day. It has been impressive to this practitioner the extent of degenerative changes that are seen in smokers on a routine basis and that a markedly deteriorated spine in a patient who is younger than the X ray is very likely a smoker or has severe pulmonary disease. Among other problems, smoking is clearly associated with increased back pain and should be eliminated. Unfortunately, this is a prevention method since no immediate negative reinforcements are perceived during smoking and, hence, the smoker continues until major damage has been done.

Considering the importance of posture and, specifically, having the ear over the point of the shoulder and this over the trochanter or pelvis to achieve a neutral position, we should minimize the stress on the spine to prevent problems. If we consider disc pressure studies, we understand that unsupported sitting has far more pressure on the disc than using a lumbar support and, thus, we should give attention to appropriate seating. Obviously, this means that some of the weight of the head and shoulders and upper trunk is transmitted through the support onto the chair and out through the spine. As we minimize the stresses in the disc, we have a better chance of preventing severe problems from chronic positions that are required for occupations, such as sitting.

When we see a patient with a frozen shoulder, we observe that the pain is essentially relieved when the motion of the shoulder has been restored. There certainly seems to be an analogy in the spine when motion is restored, pain is lessened, particularly if we increase the motion of the accompanying lower extremity. For example (Figure 21), when the hamstrings are tight, the hip is prevented from executing as great an arc of motion as would be possible with a stretched normal hamstring. Under the circumstances, bending requires more motion from the spine or increased stress than would otherwise be required. Hence hamstring stretching can be important to minimize pain in the back. Range of motion has been overemphasized by the Social Security Administration and has been a particularly significant criterion for disability in a measurement modality, which is primarily measuring motion in the hip (misinterpreted to be lumbar motion). A person can have a surgical fusion of the spine and still bend over and touch his toes. As such, the need to have motion at the hip is emphasized and also the lack of correspondence between pain and range of motion. Nonetheless, when a patient without surgical intervention can move more freely, she should have less pain. Hence, we concentrate a good deal of our effort on this aspect.

If manipulation results in temporarily decreased pain, that is a laudable goal. But this may be a relief of muscle spasms. Moving better because muscle spasm is relieved, perhaps because the facet that was the irritant under the muscles (causing them to go into spasm) now has an air bubble within it from the adjustment, may occur without a change in the range of motion of the system. Failing to increase the range of motion of muscle groups and joint capsules that are not stretched out, would suggest that this is only a temporary benefit. When the air implosion in the joint, which makes the manipulation sound in our knuckles or in our low back with the chiropractor, is resorbed, the joint may go back into spasm and be unchanged from the pre-manipulation situation. Back manipulation from a medical standpoint has a long history, which may be a consideration with analogy to the frozen shoulder. That is, when the frozen shoulder doesn't respond to physical therapy, a gradual mobilization and increased range of motion, then under a general anesthesia the patient has scar tissue broken up forcibly by manipulation. Unfortunately, the reactionary attitude of some physicians and particularly the AMA to eliminate chiropractic manipulation has prevented more widespread cooperative, collaborative, and educational investigation of manipulation and the uses of manipulation in the treatment of patients. Even though the literature does not clearly show a benefit from manipulation for chronic conditions, there are hundreds of articles including chiropractic studies which show that there is an early benefit and this seems eminently reasonable: Mobilization should be recommended rather than immobilization, such as the common bed rest that we have already discussed.

Normal spine motion includes flexion forward and extension backward. Whenever we lift something and we have the impression that it is relatively heavy, we prepare ourselves. This is automatically done by increasing intra-abdominal pressure as we strain and say, "Oomph!" Whether we do this voluntarily, or unconsciously anticipate a heavy weight, we find that stress is relieved on the spine by this maneuver, referred to as Valsalva. The Williams exercises were intended to decrease lordosis but also to strengthen the abdominal muscles, which was thought helpful to not only increase the moment arm and decrease stress on the spine but also to increase this reflex or this functional action by increasing the tone in the abdominal muscles. Certainly the abdominal muscles should be strengthened and conditioned by normal aerobic exercise, whether swimming, walking or running. In addition, the sit-ups recommended as exercises should also stretch out the muscles in the lower back, which we have previously discussed and this again reinforces the benefits of good physical conditioning and exercise.

The spine has a range of motion, which includes bending backward as well as bending forwards. From years of experience, it is clear that many patients with spine problems, and particularly with muscle limitations in their low back, are markedly limited in forward flexion. They cannot touch their toes. People who present with earlier problems and have not reached this chronic disabled state, but present for examination a first injury of a minor complaint, or even often in asymptomatic normal patients with no specific back complaints, a marked restriction is observed in their ability to bend backward or lumbar extension and in many cases fairly severely. This limitation of extension may be a result of the lack of need to achieve that position or that posture within their normal daily activities or function. Failure to

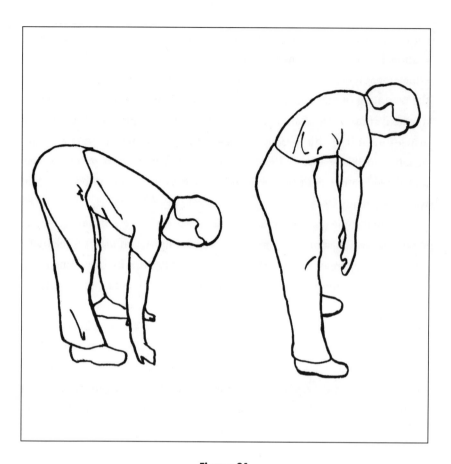

Figure 21

Forward flexion may be limited more by the hamstrings than actual spinal motion.

need to go into that posture may result in a contracture of the fascia and ligaments, which we have discussed, and, further, this is not good for the nutrition of the facet joints and the disc. The extension exercises or the MacKenzie exercises, as they have been popularized, clearly do not comprise the entirety of the program Robin MacKenzie has promoted as enhancing the motion of the facet joints far more than flexion exercises. As the facet joints move against themselves they will, hopefully, increase their range of motion and allow the brain to pick from a greater range of positions and postures while we are sitting or changing to other positions. A comfortable and pain-free position automatically can then be found by the brain, which is outside of our awareness and involuntarily function, and particularly helpful as we reduce the stiffness by increasing motion in those joints. Again, exercises such as swimming or walking can progressively loosen muscles and provide deep heat from the inside out, which is more effective than any physical therapy modality. Many studies have shown the benefit of aerobic conditioning, and I think at this time most rehabilitation professionals or reconditioning programs provide a great deal of attention in directing patients with back pain toward aerobic conditioning as part of their treatment. Although this is an indirect effect, it is not a distraction effect but truly physically treats the buildup of metabolic wastes in the muscle that are thought to provide an acidic pH (lactic acid) which is the same as causing muscle fatigue when we run a mile (if we ever run that far). This is not a matter of the physician believing that we are not truly active or not recognizing the severity of our problem, but it is known to be a beneficial, effective exercise and conditioning.

Our best program for prevention is, then, good conditioning and flexibility. This answer seems superficial and ineffective in reassuring patients who have recovered to some extent from the pain of an acute injury but continue to be stiff. Stiffness may be residual inflammation, which has not resolved, or contracture of fascia and ligaments, which have not been restored to full range of motion despite resuming normal use. Patients who do not resume normal full range of motion in their daily activities and enter into the cycle of chronic pain are likely to be permanently stiff; and, hence, our credibility at this reassurance diminishes. When physical exam shows a normal neurologic examination and only a restricted range of motion, it would then seem obvious that exercises should be prescribed to restore a

normal range of motion. This is an appropriate treatment specifically directed at the identified problem; lacking range of motion. Even though the
Social Security Administration has taken range of motion as an index of disability, it probably should be more commonly recognized that what they are
measuring is of limited relevance to the back, as it is actually hip motion;
secondly, as studies have shown, the more stiff a person is generally, the less
pain they have and more functional they may be. Patients who have total
deconditioning may be quite loose and have severe complaints of pain; so
by voluntarily attempting to demonstrate a decreased range of motion,
these patients hide the severity of their problem that is reflected in the
increased motion of unstable joints and weak muscles. Many patients seem
to feel that their residual stiffness and decreased range of motion is an index
of something bad that must be fixed, just as periodic oil changes keep our
cars from falling apart. Perhaps it should be more analogous to burning the
carbon out from having only driven in city traffic, stop and go, and up to a
blurring speed of fifteen or twenty miles an hour.

When we consider the benefits of heat and modalities such as physical therapy, we have to recognize that a hot shower or a Jacuzzi is probably equivalent in most cases to physical therapy modalities, even though
ultrasound may require a prescription; it is, nonetheless, evident that the
heat is internally applied or, from the inside out. That is, when the muscles are exercised, they will heat up, and this heat will loosen joints, cause
stiffness to diminish, and not only prevent a lot of problems but allow
normal function.

If we listen to television ads, we are probably impressed by the new
discoveries that exercises are beneficial. Obviously, the benefit of exercise
has been understood for a long time, and each of these approaches or
devices has an investor who is seeking a specific profit. Also, each of these
discoveries seems to have its own approach and a patented miracle piece of
equipment, which is directed specifically to everybody's problem. The solution in each case seems to be a specific timesaving device, which allows us
the effects of exercise without spending any time and without any inconvenience. While everyone has time demands and other needs, different
people have different problems, and we should perhaps best take the attitude that exercise in any form is going to be its own reward. This seems

somewhat more credible, and it is clearly going to be psychologically relaxing, as well as physically restoring, and will make us feel better and function more efficiently in every way. The real problem is to discover which form of exercise is for us personally enjoyable and which we are likely to continue on a basis that will become therapeutic and meaningful. This is of crucial significance because we are not dealing with a problem, we are dealing with the prevention of a problem; and, hence, we are not motivated to continue by the symptoms of the problem, but by our general interest and prudent behavior.

Prevention has been considered, and I would like to summarize it as a three-point program. First, having discussed the injuries and their treatment, we must recognize that the problem is lessened and relieved by conditioning and exercises. This initial treatment should be coupled with ergonomic analysis at the workplace to prevent further injuries, especially a repetition of the same problems; and this is the most important aspect of a prevention program from the occupational standpoint. Further, early intervention is crucial, and the most helpful component of a worker's compensation injury system is for the immediate supervisor to call the injured worker. This contact must assure the patient that he is recognized as a valued employee and that his return is sought. The supercisor should clearly assure the employee that accommodations would be made to facilitate his successful resumption of normal activities with consideration. Unfortunately, there is a lot of suffering, including back problems that occur in the home or at recreation that does not come to the attention of a physician. That is clearly in part preventable or at least modifiable by performing appropriate stretching maneuvers before athletic participation, appropriate lifting techniques for small children and laundry baskets, cervical pillows for sleeping, lumbar supports for sitting, breaks when being in a car, and so on. This has been discussed in the previous chapters and it is hoped that an increased awareness will bring us to an appreciation of the need for these techniques of lifting and concern about sitting. However, it is clear that until problems occur, many of the steps will not be implemented. Unfortunately, prevention seems to follow recovery rather than precede a problem and eliminate it.

The second level of treatment would be the prevention of the problem becoming chronic and subsequently intractable and fixed in treatment without relief of the suffering. The chronic case involves the lack of understanding of the patient and, particularly, an element of fear on the part of that patient as she presents to the doctor, but often also includes the physician's lack of appreciation of the need to avoid passive treatment and to get the patient actively involved in a rehabilitation program. Patients who continue to have pain and wait until it is completely gone before they start to rehabilitate or recondition, even after surgery or with medication, are at risk for having chronic problems. This requires a good deal of reeducation of professionals as well as patients. In the workplace, the most important preventive measure is the flexibility to make accommodations and to provide in some sense a light-duty position. That is, if the patient can remain at work performing as much as is within the physical capabilities of that patient, then the problem of becoming completely disabled or becoming a chronic case are greatly minimized. The back pain sufferer, at this point, has the natural rhythm of moving the back, of being productive, and just not being able to lift heavy things or do other activities of unacceptable strain on the back temporarily. The habit of hearing the alarm clock, arising in the morning, and traveling to work is not interrupted.

The third level of prevention would be some form of the functional restoration program, which has been described as it exists in one place in this country, but the principles of which should be incorporated in the care of all patients with back problems, and particularly, the occupational limitations. This is a case in which the patients have pain, the pain has been longstanding, but no further treatments are helpful nor can be recommended. These patients may have had multiple surgeries; they have often minimal physical findings, and clearly have a condition of chronic pain. These patients are difficult to treat because they really dictate what treatments, if any, they will accept and, more accurately, which treatments offered will be relied upon for some relief from the actual experience of pain. The problem is that the pain is preventing the patient from being functional and, as such, interferes with a patient's self-esteem, motivation, and other capabilities. These patients clearly should be able to increase their functional capacities, their enjoyment of life with self-esteem, and some measure of productivity without a commensurate increase in pain; and that is the purpose in a functional restoration program. That is, they may be able to do twice as much work without having twice as much pain, and since they were in pain without doing anything, then it is clear that they would benefit in terms of self-esteem, productivity, and physical well-being by proceeding to do more despite the pain.

It is also possible in many cases that the increase in function will lead to restoration of some normal functions, such as we have discussed disc nutrition by exercise and motion of the spine with actually an eventual decrease in pain. This may be a matter of faith, as continuing to do the work with pain over a fairly extended time does not provide pain relief in the visible immediate sense. This seems more a treatment than a mode of prevention, but it is intended as an intervention to interrupt the chronic pain cycle and to prevent its perpetuation. Having pain without being strictly disabled or preventing disability by accepting pain would perhaps be a fair statement of such a goal. But, as such, this could be viewed from a prevention standpoint.

When we consider patients who have difficulty standing up, we anticipate that these are patients with difficulties in the facet joints. The facet joints are posterior. Hence, when they are in a flexed position such as sitting, the facet joints are unloaded and the weight is on the discs. As a consequence, we would recommend extension exercises or the MacKenzie group of exercises to prevent this sort of continued pain. It should become evident after a few weeks that getting up from a chair should be less difficult and the ability to stand erect on arising from a chair facilitated. People should also be encouraged to do abdominal strengthening exercises such as the Williams exercises. These flexion exercises should strengthen the muscles, provide a hydraulic column for support, and increase the moment of effectiveness for the muscles around the spine causing less pain. Studies of unselected patients have shown that some benefit from extension exercises, and others benefit from flexion exercises, and seldom do patients actually benefit from both.

Finally, prevention should include responsibility on the part of the patient for having an active role. This, specifically, should extend to the fact that habituating narcotics are inappropriate for chronic pain; and although there is no reason to avoid taking Motrin, Advil, aspirin or other anti-inflammatories as prescribed on an indefinite basis, all narcotics, even including Darvon or codeine, should be assiduously avoided. The concept that "it is the only thing that gives me any relief" is really a cop-out. If the patient has given up on the situation and wants to be passively cured, this may be understandable but is not justifiable and it is a bad choice. I'm not saying that patients want to suffer, but the less they do to help themselves, the longer and the more they will suffer. Physicians who are quick to prescribe such medications probably also should be avoided, although patients are highly attracted to physicians overutilizing narcotics. Having then discussed methods of prevention and all the preceding discussion on what is the problem and why surgery is often not valuable, we will then shift our attention to cases in which surgery has been performed or is anticipated and discuss what should follow.

Chapter 10

POSTSURGERY

[Back surgery is] leaving more tragic human wreckage
in its wake than any other operation in history.

—DePalma, 1970

Surgery on the spine is appropriate under careful indications, which we have discussed previously; and the results can be dramatic with impressive reduction in pain and increase in function. The results for some operations are prompt, almost immediate. Other procedures involve waiting for bone to heal and that may be a slow, prolonged process. In this chapter, we would like to presume that surgery is appropriately indicated and performed in a technically correct way. Our focus will be to outline the various forms of surgery that may be performed or discussed, and the expectations of those procedures. Rehabilitation varies according to the procedure but is an integral part of the treatment and crucial for optimal recovery.

Surgery in an oversimplified lay description is either to take pressure off nerves or to stabilize the spine. Taking pressure off nerves involves a laminectomy or a discectomy in which either the bony elements, disc material, or both are removed from impinging nerves, or compressing the nerves. Spinal stabilization involves a bony fusion of some sort, with or without internal fixation or instrumentation, to hold the spine still during healing, to immobilize the flexible spinal segments, or to correct deformity which differs substantially from a fusion in place, but involves the time waiting for bone to heal.

The procedures to remove material such as disc or bone spur from nerves have a similar purpose but are quite varied. Technically, the procedures have become less invasive; and this, of course, evokes considerable interest on the part of the patients. First, some procedures are percutaneous, in which a puncture is made in the skin and instruments are inserted into the disc to remove disc material. Originally this was done quite a few years ago as a biopsy technique, but later an enzyme was developed to digest the disc material. This enzyme was chymopapain and was quickly widely used, since it was not an operation. Unfortunately, the procedure became rather controversial and has not really lived up to the expectation of being as good as an open operation. First, patients seem to have considerable muscle spasm after the procedure as well as pain, which clearly exceeds that of the customary expectation of patients who actually have the open operation. Even though this procedure uses a Band-Aid rather than a dressing for a small incision, patients are in bed longer, with more spasm in the muscles and more pain rather than less. The advantages of having no incision are rather emotional. The suggestion that no scarring occurs is not really consistent with the excess spasm and pain that is clearly an indication that the injected material clearly has influence outside of the disc itself. The enzyme is carefully placed in the disc, and modifications of the procedure have been performed, specifically, not to do a discectomy which would leave a needle tract in the disc to allow some of the enzyme to leak out; however, when you inject it with a needle there is a needle track as well. Results are inferior to an open operation, and there are patients who have severe, even fatal, allergic reactions to the material; and a significant proportion of people have scarring, and that scarring seems to lead to residual problems for which there is no remedy. Statistically, the procedure is effective and has been borne out by careful studies; but those results remain inferior, in the best hands, to actual open operation, which makes the percutaneous operation of doubtful advantage, as the open operation can be performed by any person accustomed to spinal procedures.

A subsequent procedure has been the percutaneous removal of some disc from the nucleus pulposus without the enzymatic digestion. The fifty percent of people who have severe muscle spasm requiring bed rest as opposed to people routinely being discharged the following day after open surgery, led to the development of a procedure to remove disc material mechanically rather than enzymatically. Mechanical aspiration of disc material has to be done while the patient is awake for safety, to avoid injuring the nerves, but thus becomes an outpatient procedure. A method of suction aspiration was developed to remove disc material with a rotating shaver blade, similar to what is used in joint arthroscopy. A laser was also used to vaporize some of the disc material and aspirate the smoke, which as the suction and cutting instrument which aspirated smaller pieces, these methods performed a central decompression of the disc; that is, the disc material in the center was removed to relieve the pressure. Disc material was removed as we remove meniscal material from knees with an arthroscope without the disadvantage of scar formation from leakage of the enzyme in the vicinity of the nerves and muscles and without an open operation. These procedures were effective in a strictly limited population of patients, those without any significant degeneration of the disc and with a contained herniation. That degeneration, however, is often present; and, as such, not only do we have a limited portion of the patients who would benefit from surgery as candidates for these select procedures, but also within that group there are probably some persons thought to be candidates who would actually have more signs of deterioration and, hence, be poor candidates, thus explaining the differential benefit of open surgery as having higher success rates than these procedures. If you become excessively careful in selecting patients for their percutaneous procedure, then you find yourself doing the outpatient percutaneous procedure so infrequently that the advantages become theoretical. An arthroscopic procedure was developed and incorporated the advantages of not using an enzyme, being percutaneous; but, also allowed a directed removal of disc material using a pituitary rongeur to remove disc material, that was flexible and thus could be directed toward the posterior longitudinal ligament and posterior annulus, where disc material was in proximity to the nerves. With this removal of disc fragments rather than a simple central disc decompression, there was an improvement in results to approach those of the open operation. The good results are achieved by strictly limiting the application of the procedure to the correct patient.

Finally, a minimally invasive procedure is the IDET, intradiscal electrothermy, or the annuloplasty. This procedure uses a probe that is inserted through a needle into the disc as it is gently advanced through the disc, it heats the disc to a 90-degree Centigrade temperature and this effects the structure of the donut or the annulus fibrosis. As the wall of the disc is heated to this temperature for a period of about seventeen minutes, the collagen shrinks and over time stffens. This may be done for patients who have some small herniations but is generally for patients who have difficulty sitting because of back pain which would be attributed to the instability of the disc and thus a stabilization procedure rather than a decompressive procedure. This procedure remains new, so results need to be followed over the long term to evaluate the modification of the natural history of this disease, which is produced by this procedure. It may be that patients who have a prognosis from natural history that their disc will stabilize in time, may do well; they, patients who have this problem and have thermal annuloplasty, may have a longstanding benefit or may require eventual stabilization such as a fusion and that can only be determined by long-term careful follow-up.

The microsurgical lumbar laminectomy is customarily performed by all surgeons performing spinal surgery. This procedure is performed with magnification and illumination from a microscope or using loupes for magnification directly and a headlight and has proven itself to have well over ninety percent effectiveness in appropriate candidates. There is minimum morbidity and a high success rate with appropriate patient selection. This procedure should be expected to give relief of leg pain since the pressure is removed from the nerve with one or two days in the hospital followed by two or three weeks of muscle soreness and stiffness. During the few weeks of muscle soreness from swelling and stiffness, limited sitting should be encouraged so that the patient does not stir up the muscle irritation- that is, sitting no longer than about half an hour at a time, which is long enough for meals or bathroom.

Following resolution of most of the swelling, the muscles will generally feel tight in the low back and then should be stretched out with knee-to-the-chest exercises of the Williams flexion type, as well as gradually progressing to back bends and the MacKenzie exercises so that flexibility of the spine both forward and backward is encouraged. After another two or three weeks, formal physical therapy, if necessary, can be introduced. Generally, if the patient has been active prior to the disc herniation and has not been disabled for a prolonged period, they gradually may be able to resume their activities at three or four weeks to the point of being able to return to work.

If disability has been longstanding or inactivity has resulted in loss of endurance or muscle strength, then physical therapy or even work hardening would be appropriate at that time.

Beyond the problem of discs or a spur is the generalized condition of spinal stenosis, more commonly occurring in patients who are in their sixties and not candidates to return promptly to work, particularly as they may be retired or have diminished expectations. These patients may take two or three months in resolving numbness and regaining muscle strength after a decompressive lumbar laminectomy, but generally do well just with increased walking or activities of daily living. Patients in their sixties who have extensive spinal stenosis and expect to go back to frequent bending, twisting, and lifting and have surgery for spinal stenosis are best warned in advance that those expectations may be unrealistic to avoid disappointment, but in most cases they are probably already aware of reasonable age-related restrictions.

Differentiating between the operations, the decompression relieves nerve compression or pressure on the nerves and the stabilization operations are bony fusions. We need to recognize that there is a vast difference in the magnitude of the operation, as well as the time of convalescence. When a fusion is performed, bone is customarily taken from someplace elsewhere in the body, usually a portion of the outer wall of the pelvis. This is the iliac crest and provides ample bone for grafting; although in some cases alternate material is used, either from cadavers or other substitutes which are forms of hydroxyapatite or calcium phosphate materials such as coral or other materials similar to bone which should provide a source of calcium and a lattice on which bone from the patient can grow and heal. When bone is harvested, the bed from which the bone is taken will bleed; and, hence, the operation entails blood loss considerably in excess of the laminectomy operation and the time that it takes for the bone graft to heal would be similar to a broken bone healing. This is months rather than weeks; and, generally, after a patient has a fusion either for spondylolisthesis, a developmental problem, for a fracture or a trauma, or for degenerative conditions, the expectation is that they should be healed in about a year's time and mature in two years or longer. Following this surgical procedure, particularly if metal is used as internal fixation, patients may be expected to have severe swelling at the operative site, but in many cases may have reduced pain in terms of the original preoperative pain from the internal fixation, and more pain at the bone graft donor site which was previously not painful. This is not just to trade one pain for another, but the expectation that the bone graft donor site pain will resolve and the back pain problem being treated by a fusion would not have resolved without the surgery.

The dissection and retraction of muscles necessary to get to the area where bone has to be placed for the fusion makes the fusion operation significantly more painful, longer, and results in more blood loss than a disc operation. This procedure will require a longer time in the hospital and more intensive hospital care with a possible need of blood transfusion and customarily the harvesting of a patient's own blood (autologous blood) in case transfusion is needed. The muscles remain sore for several weeks after the procedure; and sitting in an unsupported position, that is, such as in a kitchen chair or on a stool will be painful within twenty to thirty minutes because of the swollen muscles. This lasts for several weeks but the patient can start their rehabilitation early basically by walking. In addition to walking, straight leg raising in bed should be done at least ten times a day for the first several weeks to move the nerve in its bed so scarring is minimized and to start stretching the hamstrings. At some time following the procedure, stretching exercises are appropriate for the muscles that were swollen because they will tend to draw or be tight having had body fluids in them as swelling. Body fluids have proteins that act in a sense like glue to make things tight, and it is not just water and salt water that is in the muscles as the swelling. Following the range of motion, as we suggested for exercises without surgery, strengthening would follow. Beyond the muscle exercise and rehabilitation of walking patients, patients may then be advised to increase gradually their activities at home or physical therapy may be advised. Patients who have a posterior fusion with pedicle screws usually start therapy or can do some light-duty work between six and nine months and develop an ability to do more work and potentially return to full function between twelve and twenty-four months. Patients who have an interbody fusion, that is bone graft or a cage between the vertebral bodies sometimes return to function in approximately half the time of the posterior instrumented fusion.

After surgery, whether decompression or stabilization, we quickly come to grips with the fact that not all cases are uniformly and entirely successful. Clearly, a bad result after surgery is a double tragedy as the patient has not only failed to benefit from the surgery but also has undergone the procedure and endured the risks and complications associated. The good cases may be so good, particularly in terms of disc surgery, that they tell their friends to go ahead and have it done. Spine surgery carries an enormous emotional load to the preoperative patient. That is, when a patient is contemplating having their spine operated on, they are worried about what might happen. Many patients ask if they are going to be paralyzed. Despite being a common fear, we do not see patients who are paralyzed from surger; although, we frequently see patients paralyzed from a motor vehicle accident; yet this does not seem to prevent either patients from assuming roles behind the wheel of a car, or more particularly, from some of the more dangerous stunts we see every day as we drive on the highways.

The question arises when we have a surgical operation performed and the predicted or anticipated result is not obtained, as to why this would have occurred. These patients are called failed backs: and having been labeled such, consideration has been given as to the reasons underlying this failure. In many cases, we would first look at the technical procedure and see whether or not the procedure was appropriate. The first problem is, of course, when the wrong level is operated on. If you have a disc at L4-5 and operate at L3-4, you can predict a poor result: that disc will not be any better by operating on the wrong level. This is evident, but there are cases in which the correct level is operated on and pain recurs or is not relieved. We see in many of these cases recurrent disc herniations or new disc herniations, and the distinction is irrelevant when there are significant symptoms and disability. Unfortunately, this involves considerable surgical judgment because studies have shown that many of the most important and commonly used imaging tests retain the appearance of residual or recurrent discs even in cases that had a successful outcome confirming that there is relief of neural compression despite those imaging findings. We also see scar tissue which may form and cause similar symptoms; however, we have to be assured that removal of scar tissue, or neurolysis, is a fool's errand. That is, when we operate, we cause more scar and if we think we are removing scar tissue, we have deceived ourselves.

Another reason operations may fail is that the procedure was not the appropriate procedure, it was the wrong operation. This is particularly important in cases in which there is instability or the spine moves and the movement causes back pain. In cases of instability, fusion is appropriate to decrease the wobbling of the bones in the spine and the subsequent irritation of the nerve roots from motion in the spine. If a patient had a disc herniation and that disc herniation was a result of a deteriorated disc that also had abnormal motion, we would predict that removing the disc herniation may allow subsequent reherniation, or new herniation, and may fail by excessive motion to relieve the pain. Hence, we have to be careful in deciding whether to decompress the nerve root or to follow up the decompression with a fusion. Healing of a fusion takes a great deal more time, and we are reluctant to put a patient through a six-month convalescence and one-year return to work when we know that a lot of patients with a simple disc are back to work and full activity in a month to six weeks. Nonetheless, if a patient has a recurrent pain, instability needs to be carefully looked at.

When we want to avoid the extensive fusion procedure, and just try decompressing the nerve root, we may not be respecting the specific indications for these procedures and cannot expect excellent results by good luck. Many failed back surgeries have an underlying problem and the indications were not appropriate or followed completely and the results subsequently are compromised. A poor indication, certainly, is an underlying factor in many failed back surgeries. When a patient has facet disease, as we have discussed earlier, and for that problem has a disc removed which was actually asymptomatic or not causing a problem, the facet syndrome causing pain is unchanged, if not worsened by the surgical procedure. We cannot realistically expect to relieve pain all over by taking pressure off a single nerve root in a single dermatome, as single nerve roots or any surgical procedure does not affect the nerves that go all over. If a patient has knots in his muscles and the syndrome of a fibromyalgia, disc surgery is not likely to help, because this is primarily an inflammatory problem without adequate solutions and, hence, is equally unrecognized and untreated.

Some patients will have instability appropriately recognized and the fusion technically appropriately performed. But the fusion may not succeed and will not heal in 100 percent of cases. This is particularly true in smokers, with a forty percent failure rate beyond that of nonsmokers. Clearly we need to investigate the fusion with serial X rays and look for bony healing to see whether or not an arthrodesis was achieved. A fusion that has not succeeded or pathologic motion which may be present without surgery, even less than a few mm or any arbitrary criterion, may result in significant pain. Failed fusions may move very little and cause severe pain requiring repeat surgery, so the criteria or change in angulation or translation on flexion extension films may no longer apply; and for minimal motion, repeat surgery may be required.

Postoperatively and perhaps most commonly, we have a situation where the pressure on the nerve is relieved. If a fusion is required, and the fusion has succeeded, then at this point the surgeon can say, "There is nothing more that I can do." As the captain of the ship, we may feel that it is incumbent upon the surgeon to do something but, in fact, surgery is not part of that plan. Rehabilitation should be directed independently and objectively by a specialist in that area in consultation with the surgeon regarding the specific case being treated. The MRI has shown that the nerves are not compressed and are seen better than previous studies. With gadolinium, contrast for the MRI, we can effectively evaluate whether a specific nerve root has disc material compressing it or whether there is scar encasing the nerve as would be expected after surgery. The scar tissue should not be touched and will not help the patient; the disc herniation may require another operation. In any case, the basic premise after an operation is that surgical options are over.

When further surgery is not available, the patient needs to learn to cope with the situation as it exists. Many times as coping mechanisms proliferate and the patient becomes more able to deal with the problem, we see that the pain diminishes and recovery, at least partially, will progress. After surgery in uncomplicated cases, we sometimes see a failure of complete benefit from lack of postoperative exercise and rehabilitation. Rehabilitation after spine surgery should consist at least of some minimal exercises after three or four weeks of relative inactivity and avoidance of prolonged sitting which stirs up the muscles and causes swelling and recurrent pain. As we proceed through this time schedule of recovery, flexibility exercises need to be reintroduced and followed by muscle strengthening or work hardening if heavy lifting is anticipated. This time schedule is delayed in the case of a fusion as opposed to a disc operation, but equally essential that healing proceed before activities can be resumed. Recent advances in spinal fixation have allowed fusions with pedicle screws and rods or plates, and without the large braces that were customary after fusions, and which probably provided a limited level of immobilization consistent with the high number of repeat surgeries which had been required and were associated with fusion operations. Studies have shown that an objective analysis fails in many cases to demonstrate the result of a fusion. That is, the results in patients who had a failed fusion were about equal to patients who had successful fusions. As a consequence, it is difficult for the surgeon to say to the patient, "Your problems will be relieved after the fusion is solid," if the surgeon is aware of the statistics. However, when a patient is fused and has internal fixation, there will be immediate relief of some of the problems and without the prolonged immobilization of the brace to create other noncompensated problems. My opinion is that the outlook is good for an improved success rate with spine surgery and, particularly, with fusions. Surgeons would do well to heed the advice that they should advertise less pain rather than no pain.

The bottom line is that of patients who have surgery, many have had definitive treatment and there may be a residual. The patient will have to learn to cope with what is left over and understand that even if there is still pain, the priority of doing the best for themselves and their family in the future rather than thinking that they are going to get even for the insult of the lawyers and rehabilitation nurse and compensation system is really a self-destructive attitude and has to be avoided. Residual pain may be from sources such as myofaciitis, facet syndrome, and other sources. As the surgery has relieved the primary problem, they are now faced with dealing with the associated situation. Coping with it is best performed through a pain clinic or an experience with a comprehensive program and with resumption gradually of all activities with an attempt to actively take control of the process and resume being normal. Becoming normal or returning to normal activities is primarily a matter of the will. The determined patient is more likely to get back to normal than the passive patient who is waiting for the doctor to declare that they have healed and that they are fine. Patients after surgery, of course, have scar tissue and removal of scar tissue cannot be done with an operation. The operation will only cause more scar tissue and will inflame the present scar tissue. Again, this is a matter in which patients need to learn to cope. They may need distraction techniques such as a TENS unit which provides a buzz that gets the attention of the brain and takes focus away from the pain. They may require injections or implanted stimulators, but in any case, they really have to deal with the situation as it is, as the last resort of having had surgery is no longer a resort.

Patients who have had a relatively good result may have other problems and this situation is not uncommon. For example, a patient may have an injury requiring surgery on the spine and, while recovering from back surgery on the spine, may have a neck problem or some other situation arise complicating their recovery, complicating their insurance coverage and frustrating their treating physician. Unfortunately, this situation is not uncommon, but the solution is relatively simple. The patient needs to recognize that this is a problem, that there are multiple possible insurance carriers which we feel are liable, and even though they will all deny payment and expect the other to cover medical costs and wages, we have a need for the patient to look beyond the delay in settlement, to look beyond the denial and insults from the insurance carrier, and to look beyond their disability, and to again take the situation into their hands and become actively involved in looking at whatever options may be available to them. That is, a patient who has had surgery and cannot go back into the coal mines or cannot return to heavy lifting needs to, as early as possible, look into further vocational training, further education, or whatever options are available to her for the rest of her life. As we see more and more workers who have difficulty with heavy lifting and other problems, it seems entirely inappropriate that a person who is no longer able to lift 100 pounds dead weight off the floor should be permanently and totally disabled for life, as there are certainly other jobs they can undertake. It is, however, the pent up rage and anger of a patient and a result of the treatment received that makes him a chronic disability patient in so much pain that he is unable to do anything. The solution is to concentrate on the things that he can do and for him to accept the need for his own motivation, which in the long run will be in his best interests, and to see what he can do rather than what he can't do. This is the basic philosophy used for patients who have disabilities; that is, to see themselves as able to do some things and to enable them to do more.

Chapter 11

PRODUCTIVITY

When men are employed, they are best contented;
for on the days they worked, they are good-natured
and cheerful, and, with a consciousness of having done
a good day's work, they spend the evening jolly;
but on our idle days, they were mutinous and quarrelsome.

—Benjamin Franklin

Patients with low back pain are able to do many things and unable to do others. It has been shown, and is a premise underlying rehabilitation programs, that on many occasions people can be restored by progressively increasing exercise resistance or activities with endurance of pain complaints. That is, as they do more, they have more pain, but not in a correlated fashion; that is, they don't have twice the pain with twice the work, they have slightly more pain with much more work, and eventually they are doing a great deal more and have pain, whereas they previously had pain doing nothing at all. Consequently, resumption of activity is an essential part of the rehabilitation process.

Success in our endeavors is a matter of focusing on our goals. Certainly if our goal is to be relieved of pain, we have absolutely no success with having substantial relief of pain which would allow us to resume activities essentially the same as prior to the problem. This is a matter of lack of focus and almost certain failure can be predicted if we take a nonnegotiable position of demanding absolute relief of pain. Unless we have something clearly in mind we are attempting to do or an appropriate focus for our activities and subsequently organize toward achieving that goal, we are really aiming at nothing and that is something we can by default (nothing!) achieve.

The problem that seems to be rampant in our society, where we may have previously been litigating and fighting a battle over a car accident, having long since fixed the car and resumed our activities, is now the problem of our health costs and disability. As we are unable to go on with our activities because of this disability, we are left fixed in place or stalemated because of the clouds of various issues of fault and sometimes even retribution or getting even. The problem is that you fail to recognize the options that are available and stubbornly refuse to go on. When we seek to live in the past and get even, we are really going to become losers, however well we fight the battle. Henry Wadsworth Longfellow pointed out that we really see ourselves in terms of our plans and what we would like to do, whereas others see us in terms of our accomplishments. When we are litigating, we may or may not find the court sympathetic to our claim for loss of opportunity, our inability to do the things that we feel we would have done, and if we succeed, we win the lottery; if we fail, we lose any hope for salvage and, when we cease to struggle, we submit to some impairment, a decreased capacity to overcome that problem.

I have been impressed in practice that there really are some patients who predict a bad result. "Everything goes wrong for me. I take twice as long to heal as anyone else," and so forth. This does not fit into the medical mind, as we know the predictability of the healing of a skin incision, and we remove a disc, bad appendix, etc., with the same instruments and the same techniques. It is peculiar that patients who expect to do poorly and consider themselves slow healers and often do have less than the usual good result, may nonetheless be the most grateful patients because they appreciate having someone care for them. Their problem may not be an impressive good result to the surgeon who expects more, but to them with their diminished expectations, they are pleased that in their opinion, for them, it was really good. The bottom line is that we are not all athletes, and that we are not all the same. Some of us would like to get straight A's and others would be content to pass when we were in school. Some of us at work would like to get promoted at a record rate. Others would like to put in our time and get to retirement. When we consider spine problems, we need more and more to recognize that spine problems occur for all people without distinction, both the motivated and the unmotivated, and that a real, painful stimulus is almost always present in these backs. In no way would we deny that there is a source of pain; but we clearly see that patients who are motivated, who get actively involved in their back pain just as they do in all of their other problems, overcome the problem, return to productivity, and realize their expectations. These patients can be identified before proposed surgery.

The purpose of this chapter is not to say that there are good patients and bad patients, but that there is a role for the patient: to take matters into his or her own hands and that attitude will significantly benefit that patient. As a physician, I feel an obligation to be an advocate of the patient, not only because of the Hippocratic Oath (which is no longer mandatory), but because I represent the patient's last resort. If I find that the patient is able to go to work, and affix my signature to such a release, but the patient finds the job situation intolerable, they subsequently will find that they have lost their job, their hope, their wages, and they really have nowhere else to turn. They can find another physician who may be more sympathetic, but they will be faced with my declaration of their fitness for work, which may not only haunt them, but may be adjudicated to be correct to their detriment. Although I would frankly prefer not to raise the issue, I am aware of patients who have committed suicide when their physician became unsupportive, because they lost their last hope in terms of their compensation claim or medical condition. This is clearly not a matter of insincerity, of mental health problems, or of malingering, but of inability to cope with the situation. This is the reality of which we have to be aware. Further, a well-known spine surgeon who gave excellent lectures to medical students, was shot by one of his patients, who also murdered his wife. This attack followed the surgeon's release of the patient to light duty, and pressure by the compensation system to get the bum back to work.

Employers are dealing with economic survival and the need to make a profit in a competitive world, so the issues of patient dignity and compassion cannot be a priority in business. This is an area in which the physician has a key role, which cannot be forgotten, and which may need to be reminded to the employer and insurance carrier that these are human injuries, not bent fenders, although there is an analogy in the insurance treatment. Although this may seem to go without saying, it is diminishingly part of the awareness of those who deal with the insurance companies, their attorneys, the patient's attorneys, and read the reports from the all-knowing technological equipment such as MRI, CT scan, and computer results from exercise machines. Unfortunately, the most important information and the most accurate and valuable is often from the physical exam performed by the physician. This information, particularly pain complaints that are subjective and not objective, may be discounted by the insurance carrier indifferent to their position, their economic interest, and their hired experts. What is considered in court are the facts and this emphasizes black-and-white objective findings, despite the fact that patients come with pain. The authority of the MRI, even though the MRI has a one-third false positive rate, is probably inordinate because it is an objective finding. Worst, the physician may increasingly rely upon these technological results. Rather than a simple and far less expensive but more important result of the simple exam, the physician will be unable to help many patients who may enter the spiral of confusion and chronic disability.

Nonetheless, I feel it necessary to say that many patients do not achieve the result possible for them, and I am unable to affect their result positively, because it really has come down to a matter of their participation. But this is a difficult point to make without having the patient sense that I am failing to continue to be supportive of his individual case. This was the purpose of the chapter on passivity, that the patient not only needs to be actively involved in doing the exercise but also, mostly, in deciding what the goals and focus of one's activities are so one can achieve the best result for oneself.

Productivity is the description of what we are doing without regard to any handicaps that might be in place. It is interesting to see in the literature regarding patients with spinal cord injury that, in fact, a majority, if not a surprisingly large number of over ninety percent of patients in some studies who are paralyzed, return to productive employment. The most important thing to recognize is that patients who are paralyzed know that they cannot walk again and they have accepted the situation. They are not nor ever will be as they were and, thus, they have to focus on what they have and what they want subsequently. Recognizing this fact and perhaps accepting the situation whether they are fully compensated and whether it was fair or reasonable, they have to use all their resources to achieve maximum ultimate function for their future. Patients who have a back problem and perhaps have a little numbness may be worried about progression, but yet there is no hidden population of people who had a little numbness, who subsequently became paralyzed and, hence, there is no basis for a fear that the numbness will not only progress but become a serious problem such as paralysis. On the other hand, if we look at the number of patients who are paralyzed and return to productive function, perhaps this would be the greatest reassurance we could give, that if it got bad and paralyzed them, the results would suggest that they would be far better off from a work standpoint. Perhaps I am being facetious, but patients with back problems should identify their goals, and if their goals are to have people sympathetic or to make accommodations because of their dependency or if their goal is truly have people interested following the social question, "How are you?" by an enumeration of all their pains and ills and suffering, then they should recognize that they are not going to be as productive as they can be or they should be. I doubt that anyone would state as such that these are their goals and it seems a waste of professional talent to say that we need psychological counseling to come to the conclusion that our actual behavior is reflecting these goals rather than the stated goals.

Without being introspective or being critical toward physicians, we clearly need to recognize medically that, despite patient lack of acceptance and unpopularity, our goal and focus must be on assisting the patient to get over the disability, which is the true problem, rather than just focusing on the back pain. If we are distracted by the constant repetitive vociferous articulated desire, "Doc, just help me with the pain," then we are distracted from recognizing the patient's problem as being inability to do things rather than the hurt. We may have pain from which we are recovering and go to work anyway. We may be unable to sleep, as in my case when my teenage son takes the car and goes to the movies with his friends: I have no pain but I can't sleep, as do many people who are unable to cope with their back pain disability problem and use the lack of sleep as the description of the severity of pain, who are resistant to being described as having difficulty coping, but truly this is the problem. For these individuals we need to focus on what we can do, what we are unable to do, and look forward in time, setting goals. In fact, goal setting as an objective or as a discipline should be taught as part of an effective rehabilitation program.

The average worker who recalls the negligence, in their opinion, of the employer in terms of leaving the grease spill that they slipped in on the floor, doesn't want to hear about how they need to set goals. They want to be compensated for a tort. The problem in terms of accomplishment is that the concern is focused on last season's problems. Chinese proverbs have suggested that failures are the mother of learning, or as one of my pathology professors stated it, repetition is a mother of learning, but mistakes are the mother-in-law. Another Chinese proverb suggests an important perspective, that our lack of success will allow us to achieve greater things than previously. When we have been defeated on the sports field, we regroup. We may seek to have a building year in terms of acquiring talent for our team. We may get a new coach, we may develop new plays, new strategies, but we go forward. If we have an appeal over an umpire's call, we don't let that conflict harm our next game; and during the course of a sports event, we cannot let a bad call early in the game lead us to defeat ourselves by allowing that to fester and detract us from the sportsmanship and desire to win that is part of our game strategy.

Productivity is also part of the adventure that we once may have enjoyed when we were developing through high school and starting our careers and considered ourselves to have many options. At some point, we developed complacency, have many years in with the company, have children whose tuition and expenses we need to pay, our mortgage to satisfy, and other obligations that leave us in a position in which we are not able to make changes or consider other occupations we might enjoy more, but we really work for the paycheck. Unfortunately, some companies may not succeed and their employees suffer. Whether international competition affects the availability of domestic jobs, whether the product being made is no longer in demand, or even if it is because an individual has sustained a work injury preventing them from returning to their particular job, we then are confronted with a problem for which social services in terms of the worker's compensation system is available. But this needs to be viewed as a matter not for us to get as much as we can with every reason to collect our entitlement, but for us to do what we can (returning to the idea of the chapter on passivity), so that we can move forward and view the subsequent many years as a success, using the losses incurred as a stepping-stone for further accomplishment. Technology has caused many changes in our society. Around the twentieth century it was commented that the population of New York City could never exceed one half million persons because, after all, where would they keep all the horses? I recall discussing this with a chairman of an orthopedic department whose immediate response was that today we could calculate how deep the horse manure would be when we got to one million. This is, indeed, the achievement of technology in computer simulations and calculations. Nonetheless, the simple fact is that horses are still around, but so are cars; and even though we may be worse off by having the population of New York exceeding one half a million, the facts are clear that it does exceed that number greatly. While adults encourage their children to get an education to have the ability to perform a variety of tasks, adults making this recommendation because of their own feeling of being locked in to their present position, and need to view their options with greater flexibility, if they should become patients with back problems or claimants in the worker's compensation system.

Our purpose here is not to go into the ten secret steps of success or to promote any particular method or plan. As a multitude of books are available on the subject of self-help and dealing with chronic problems. But our purpose is to suggest the connection between disability from a back problem or, in fact, other problems and the need for a comprehensive rehabilitation program, which we have discussed at many points during this text, but which at sometimes is clearly necessary, but is limited as it only functions efficiently with the appropriate attitude of cooperation on the part of the patient. My role as a physician is not only to recommend the appropriate program but to seek to help the patient learn, to some extent within the time available, the need for that program and how it is going to help them as an individual. This would be an extended discussion for many patients, and, hence, this assembled text of information. Hopefully with knowledge there is increased strength and with increased strength there will be satisfaction and accomplishment.

LIST OF ILLUSTRATIONS